PHARMACY COLLEGE ADMISSION TEST (PCAT)

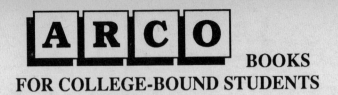

ARCO BOOKS
FOR COLLEGE-BOUND STUDENTS

COLLEGE ENTRANCE

ACT: American College Testing Program
ACT English Workbook
ACT Math Workbook
College Board Achievement Test in English Composition
College Board Achievement Test in Mathematics: Level I
College Board Achievement Test in Mathematics: Level II
College Board Achievement Test in Spanish
Cram Course for the ACT
Cram Course for the SAT
Nursing School Entrance Examinations
PCAT: Pharmacy College Admissions Tests
Preparation for the SAT: Scholastic Aptitude Test
SAT Math Workbook
SAT Verbal Workbook
SuperCourse for the ACT
SuperCourse for College Board Achievement Tests
SuperCourse for the SAT

ADVANCED PLACEMENT

Advanced Placement Examination in American History
Advanced Placement Examination in Biology
Advanced Placement Examination in Chemistry
Advanced Placement Examination in Computer Science
Advanced Placement Examination in English Composition and Literature
Advanced Placement Examination in European History
Advanced Placement Examination in Mathematics
Preparation for the CLEP: College-Level Examination Program

COLLEGE GUIDES

The American Film Institute Guide to College Courses in Film and Television
College Admissions: A Handbook for Students and Parents
College Applications Step by Step
College Financial Aid
College Survival
Lovejoy's College Guide
The Right College
200 Most Selective Colleges

AVAILABLE AT BOOKSTORES EVERYWHERE

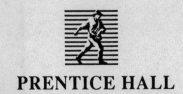

PRENTICE HALL

ARCO

PHARMACY COLLEGE ADMISSION TEST (PCAT)

Dick R. Gourley, Pharm. D
Professor of Clinical Pharmacy and Dean of
College of Pharmacy
The University of Tennessee, Memphis

CONTRIBUTING EDITORS

Greta A. Gourley, B.S.N., M.S.N., Ph. D.

BIOLOGY
Bradford Jensen, Ph. D

MATHEMATICS AND CHEMISTRY
Patricia A. Cleveland, M.S., Ph. D.

and

Ariff Rose, B. Pharm., M.S.

Prentice Hall
New York • London • Toronto • Sydney • Tokyo • Singapore

Second Edition

Prentice Hall General Reference
15 Columbus Circle
New York, NY 10023

An Arco Book

Arco, Prentice Hall, and colophons are
registered trademarks of Simon & Schuster, Inc.

Manufactured in the United States of America

2   3   4   5   6   7   8   9   10

Library of Congress Cataloging-in-Publication Division

Gourley, D.R.H.
    Pharmacy college admission test (PCAT) / Dick R. Gourley;
contributing editors, Greta A. Gourley; biology, Bradford Jensen;
mathematics and chemistry, Patricia A. Cleveland and Ariff Rose.
—2nd ed.
    p. cm.
Includes biographical references.
ISBN 0-13-656232-9
1. Pharmacy colleges—United States—Entrance examinations—Study guides.
I. Gourley, Greta A. II. Title.
[DNLM: 1. College Admission Test. 2. Pharmacy—examination questions. QV 18 G716p]
RS105.G67   1991
615'.1'071173—dc20
DNLM / DLC
for Library of Congress   91-4537
                                              CIP

CONTENTS

Part Four: PCAT Review

PART ONE

PHARMACY PRACTICE

Introduction to the Profession of Pharmacy: Historical Perspective

The origins of the profession of pharmacy can be traced to the time of ancient Babylonia–Assyria, Egypt, and Greece (approximately 3000 B.C.) Although very little is known of pharmacy at this time, fragments of knowledge provide some clues. The word *pharmacy* and its derivatives can be traced this far back and to some degree explain the meaning of the Greek word *pharmakon*. Opinions are divided as to whether there were pharmacists in ancient Egypt or, rather, "physician assistants" who specialized in the preparation of pharmaceuticals.

Originally, pharmacy was the work of priests, but it then became a part of the function of lay medical practitioners, who combined medicine and pharmacy. The birth of the European professional pharmacy occurred some time around 1240 A.D. when the German Emperor Frederick II issued "an edict that was to be the Magna Charta of the profession of pharmacy" (see Kramer and Urdang's *History of Pharmacy*, Lippincott, Philadelphia, 1963.) As medicine and pharmacy grew and matured, the pharmacist became responsible for the preparation and dispensing of medications, and in European societies became known as an apothecary (also around 1240 A.D.). The physician became responsible for diagnosing and treating illness.

Educationally, pharmacy has evolved from an apprenticeship that did not require any formal education to a sophisticated professional degree program. The standard dictionary definition of pharmacy is "the art or practice of preparing, preserving, compounding, and dispensing drugs." Traditionally, the pharmacist has been thought of as a compounder and dispenser of medications; however, with the advances of twentieth-century technology, the pharmacist has taken on new roles and responsibilities. Traditional pharmacist roles include the following:

- Dispensing medications
- Compounding medications
- Storing and purchasing medications
- Advising patients and other health care providers on drugs

Since the 1960s the pharmacy profession has moved toward a more patient-oriented practice rather than a product-oriented one. This is partly a response to the increasing numbers of new drug products that have appeared on the market, and the growing need for patient information about those drugs. Patients have become more aggressive in their quest for information about the medications and drug regimens prescribed for them. The new clinical patient-oriented roles of the pharmacist include the following:

1. **Counseling patients**—Discussing the correct way to store and take the medication, as well as answering questions about the patient's disease.

2. **Monitoring**—Observing the patient's drug therapy to assure that the drug is accomplishing its purpose, and to assure that no side effects or adverse drug reations are occurring.

3. **Providing pharmacokinetic consultations**—Providing information to physicians on drug absorption, excretion, and drug metabolism on specific drugs. This allows for individualized dosing, which assures optimal drug therapy results.

4. **Relating drug information**—Providing this knowledge to physicians, nurses, other pharmacists, dentists, and other health care providers.

5. **Prescribing**—Pharmacists have traditionally had the responsibility of recommending over-the-counter drugs to patients; however, over the past several years there have been changes in pharmacy practice laws in several states that have promoted the pharmacist as a prescriber under protocol for certain diseases. Florida has passed a law which allows pharmacists to prescribe a third class of drugs, apart from physician-prescribed and over-the-counter drugs.

Here is how one prominent study of pharmacy summarizes the present and future roles of the pharmacist:

Pharmacy should be defined basically as a system which renders a health service by concerning itself with knowledge about drugs and their effects upon man and animal. Pharmacy generates knowledge about drugs, acquires relevant knowledge from the biological, chemical, physical, and behavorial sciences; it tests, organizes, and applies that knowledge. Pharmacy translates a substantial portion of that knowledge into drug products and distributes them widely to those who require them. Pharmacy knowledge is disseminated to physicians, pharmacists, other health care providers, and to the general public to the end that drug knowledge and products may contribute to the health of individuals and to the welfare of society. The knowledge system of pharmacy through its therapeutic use is a substantial and significant segment of health care in the United States.*

If you wish to read more about the pharmacist's responsibilities relating to pharmaceutical aspects of drug therapy in contemporary pharmacy practice, we recommend Kahlman and Schlegel's article "Standards of Practice for the Profession of Pharmacy", *American Pharmacy*, Vol. 19, No. 3, page 31, 1979. Other suggested readings include:

1. "Pharmacy in the 21st Century Conference: Executive Summary," *The Consultant Pharmacist*, April 1990, Vol. 5, No. 4, pages 226–233.

2. Manasse, Henri R., Jr., "Medication Use in an Imperfect World," American Society of Hospital Pharmacists, 1989.

3. Hepler, C.D., "The Third Wave in Pharmaceutical Education: The Clinical Movement," *American Journal Pharmacy Education*, No. 51, pages 369–384, 1987.

4. Cocolas, G.H., "Pharmacy in the 21st Century Conference: Executive Summary, *American Journal Pharmacy Education*, Winter, 1989.

Career Opportunities

Since the 1960s, pharmacy education and practice has undergone significant changes that will continue to unfold in the foreseeable future. Pharmacy is still evolving, even though it is an old and honored profession. Job opportunities exist in a variety of areas including, but not limited to, independent community pharmacy, hospital pharmacy, chain store pharmacy, the pharmaceutical industry, government, geriatric pharmacy

*Pharmacists For the Future. The Report of the Study Commission on Pharmacy. Ann Arbor; Health Administration Press, 1975.

services, clinical practice in a variety of specialty areas, nuclear pharmacy, and in interdisciplinary fields that involve other health professional areas.

As you can readily see, job opportunities are varied. Individuals who complete either a bachelor of science in pharmacy (B.S.) or a doctor of pharmacy degree (Pharm. D.) have many choices available to them. Postgraduate education also offers an excellent opportunity for continuing one's education and building upon the basics of pharmacy education. The following are brief descriptions of the career opportunities available to individuals who complete the basic requirements for pharmacy licensure.

Community Pharmacy

Community pharmacy is becoming a practice that provides a variety of health services to patients. In addition to having responsibility for the distribution of drugs to patients, the pharmacist is also responsible for educating the patient about medications. Because of the ever-increasing amount of pharmaceutical knowledge and information, professionals in other areas of health care are turning more frequently to pharmacists for advice and assistance. Pharmacists contribute information that is helpful in selecting the best drug therapy for a patient and can help physicians monitor the patient's progress. Pharmacists must detect possible adverse reactions patients may have to drugs and interactions that may occur between drugs. They have the opportunity and responsibility of advising patients in their use of nonprescription drugs. In addition, they must make recommendations to patients and other health professionals for avoiding problems with drug use.

The practice of community pharmacy is also a business. In addition to their patient care activities, pharmacists must also manage people, resources, and time. The opportunities for community involvement and establishing long-term relationships with patients make community practice exciting. Opportunities are available in rural and metropolitan areas of the country, as well as in a variety of settings, such as apothecaries, chain stores, and independent community pharmacies.

Hospital Pharmacy

Pharmacists in hospitals supervise the distribution of drugs to patients. In addition, they are increasingly assuming responsibility for patient education on drug therapy, taking the medication histories of admitted patients, assisting in monitoring the drug regimens of patients, making patient rounds with physicians and nurses to provide drug information, participating in cardiac codes, and providing pharmacokinetic and therapeutic consultations to physicians. Pharmacists serve as consultants to other health professionals on drug therapy, and in many hospitals conduct in-service education programs for other health professionals on issues related to the use of drugs. In addition, some pharmacists may work in a nuclear pharmacy preparing the various radiopharmaceuticals used in programs of chemotherapy and various testing procedures. Decentralization of pharmacy services has expanded the role of hospital pharmacists and added clinical responsibilities. Hospital pharmacists specialize in a variety of areas, including administration, pediatrics, medicine, surgery, oncology, psychiatry, nutrition, and drug information.

Pharmaceutical Industry

Many pharmaceutical firms employ pharmacists in research, product development, quality control, clinical research, sales, marketing, management and other areas. Pharmacists, as well as other scientists, are responsible for testing and controlling the production of drugs. Pharmacists also work in regulatory affairs, dealing with the Food and Drug Administration (FDA), as well as in professional affairs. The professional affairs area includes working with other pharmacists, physicians, and other health care providers, and the general public.

Once pharmaceuticals have been manufactured, they must be marketed. Pharmacists therefore also serve as medical service representatives (the sales force of the pharmaceutical industry). These representatives call on physicians, dentists, veterinarians, pharmacies (hospital, community, extended-care facilities, government agencies), and nurses to explain the uses and merits of the products that their firms manufacture.

Clinical research and product development is a relatively new area within the pharmaceutical industry. Numerous pharmacists are employed to monitor and control clinical research in this field.

Another area of industry that employs pharmacists concerns drug information. These pharmacists provide drug information about the companies' products to health care providers (including pharmacists, nurses, and physicians) and to the general public. They also serve as a resource for sales and marketing forces.

Government Pharmacy Practice

Many pharmacists work for public health departments on a state or local level, as well as for the federal government. In the FDA, pharmacists work with physicians and other health care providers in assessing good manufacturing practices and the efficacy of new drug products. In the United States Public Health Service, pharmacists are employed as either institutional pharmacy practitioners, administrators, or clinic pharmacists. Pharmacy positions are also available in other governmental agencies, such as the National Institutes of Health. There are also opportunities in the armed forces, each of which has pharmacists that are commissioned officers. Pharmaceutical services are provided in health care facilities or on various bases in the United States and abroad.

Nuclear Pharmacy

Nuclear pharmacy is a unique specialty area within pharmacy. Individuals who specialize in nuclear pharmacy work with radioactive medications and diagnostic agents and their preparation. Pharmacists must be certified to work with radioactive materials and generally a postgraduate course is required. Pharmacy students may take electives in nuclear pharmacy in schools of pharmacy that offer such programs. Postgraduate courses may cover the minimum requirement of two hundred hours of work or may include graduate course work leading to a M.S. degree or even to a Ph.D.

Geriatric Pharmacy Practice

The fastest growing segment of the population is the group aged 65 and older. In 1880, they represented 3 percent of the population, while in 1980, they represented 11.3 percent of the population. By the year 2010, they will be 22.5 percent of the population. Geriatric patients have more chronic diseases and therefore use more over-the-counter medications and prescription medications than any other age group. Because of their medication needs and the unique problems of drug therapy in the elderly, geriatric pharmacy practice has emerged as a specialty. Such a practitioner provides therapeutic consultation, patient counseling and education, and in-service education to nursing staffs of extended-care facilities as well as therapeutic consultations to physicians on the drug therapy of the elderly. Dispensing services are also required for these facilities. This is a new area of practice and one that offers a rewarding and challenging career.

Clinical Practice Specialty Areas

During the past twenty years a clinical practice of pharmacy has developed that focuses on the provision of therapeutics to patients in specific areas. For example, there are pharmacists who are now practicing in the specialty areas of pediatrics, oncology, psychiatry, critical care medicine, pharmacokinetics, geriatrics, pulmonary medicine, and infectious disease, to mention a few. These practitioners provide these services to patients in hospitals and/or clinic situations. In most cases, to practice in these specialty areas, besides the basic entry-level degree for the profession, you will need a residency or fellowship. The majority of people entering these practices today have a Pharm.D. degree and either a specialty residency or fellowship.

Summary

The profession of pharmacy is a dynamic and changing one and should you select pharmacy as your career goal, you will find it rewarding and challenging. The areas of practice are so many and so varied, that each person should be able to find a field suitable to his or her particular or skills and interests.

PART TWO

PHARMACY EDUCATION

American Council on Pharmaceutical Education

Pharmacy colleges are accredited by the American Council on Pharmaceutical Education (ACPE). The ACPE was established in 1932 and is the national accrediting agency in pharmacy recognized by the Secretary of Education, United States Department of Education, and the Council on Post-Secondary Accreditation (COPA). The council is also a member of the Council of Specialized Accrediting Agencies. The ACPE is an autonomous agency whose membership is derived through the American Association of Colleges of Pharmacy (AACP), the American Pharmaceutical Association (APHA), and the National Association of Boards of Pharmacy (NABP), with three members each appointed by the respective associations. In addition, there is one member appointed from the American Council on Education (ACE). Thus, there are ten members of the Council. In addition, a panel of public representatives serves in an advisory capacity to the council and provides for public contribution to its proceedings. The American Foundation for Pharmaceutical Education provides major financial support for the council's general activities. The AACP, APHA, and NABP also provide annual support to sustain the council's activities. A list of accredited degree programs, published annually, is available from the ACPE office on request (American Council on Pharmaceutical Education, One East Wacker Drive, Chicago, Illinois 60601).

Students must graduate from a college or school of pharmacy that is accredited by the American Council on Pharmaceutical Education to be eligible to take the NABPLEX (National Association of Boards of Pharmacy Licensure Examination) given by the state board of pharmacy in their state. This is the exam that licenses pharmacist to practice. Each state gives the examination with the exceptions of California and Louisiana, which give their own examinations. You should contact each state to determine when and how often the board examination is given, and if you have other questions concerning the requirements of that state.

Institutions and Programs*

There are 74 colleges and schools of pharmacy in the United States. Seventy-two have accredited first professional degree programs and two have programs in precandidate accreditation status. A few Pharm.D. programs have not yet been accredited by the American Council on Pharmaceutical Education. Twenty programs are in private institutions and 54 are in publicly supported universities. There are three independent, free-standing pharmacy schools, all private. The remaining 71 schools are university affiliated. Thirty-five schools of pharmacy are part of an academic health center campus. Sixty-three schools offer the B.S. in pharmacy. Twenty-two schools offer the Pharm.D. as the first professional degree; at 11 of these schools the Pharm.D. is the only first professional degree program. Forty schools offer the Pharm.D. as a post B.S. degree. Fifty-three schools have graduate programs in pharmacy at the Ph.D. level and 52 at the M.S. level. There are 3,022 full-time pharmacy faculty members at the 74 schools and colleges of pharmacy.

*Figures are from the October 1989 report of the American Association of Colleges of Pharmacy.

Twelve Schools Offer the Pharm.D. as the Only Professional Degree

University of Arizona
University of California, San Francisco
University of the Pacific (California)
University of Southern California
Mercer University (Georgia)
Idaho State University

University of Illinois at Chicago
University of Michigan
University of Nebraska
University of North Dakota
Campbell University (North Carolina)
University of Tennessee

Twenty-Two Pharmacy Schools Offer the Option of Either a Pharm.D. or B.S. as the Entry-Level Degree

Samford University (Alabama)
Howard University (District of
  Columbia)
Florida A&M University
Southeastern College of Pharmaceutical
  Sciences (Florida)
University of Florida
University of Georgia
Purdue University (Indiana)
University of Kansas
University of Kentucky
Xavier University of Louisiana
University of Maryland

University of Minnesota
St. Louis College of Pharmacy
  (Missouri)
University of Missouri–Kansas City
Creighton University (Nebraska)
Rutgers University (New Jersey)
University of North Carolina
Philadelphia College of Pharmacy and
  Science (Pennsylvania)
University of South Carolina
University of Texas at Austin
University of Utah
Virginia Commonwealth University

Pharmacy Students

Pharmacy student enrollment has ranged from 114 to 1,136 students per school in recent years. Schools report an application to enrollment rate of about 2.2:1, and enrollment has been rising since the mid 1980s. There were nearly 30,000 full-time students enrolled in pharmacy professional programs in 1989; about 25,000 students were enrolled in B.S. programs, and more than 4,000 were enrolled in six-year Pharm.D. programs. About 60 percent of the total students were women and over 11 percent were minority students. There were also about 2,500 full-time graduate students enrolled in Ph.D. and M.S. programs in pharmacy.

The average age of students applying to pharmacy programs has been rising (it was slightly over 22 in 1989), and so has the grade point average of those students. Projections are that the grade point average for enrollees in pharmacy programs will continue to move upward from the 3.13 of last year's entering class, and that colleges and schools will be able to be increasingly selective in offering places to the growing numbers of better qualified applicants.

Special Section: Trends and Developments in Pharmacy Education

Curriculum Evolution: What Progress Have We Made?

Dick R. Gourley
College of Pharmacy, University of Tennessee, 874 Union Avenue, Memphis, TN 38163

The following pages discuss changes that have taken place in the pharmacy curriculum over the last twenty years. They have been adapted from an article that appeared in the American Journal of Pharmacy Education, *Vol. 53, Winter 1989. (Reprinted with permission.)*

Introduction

In preparing for this discussion today, a number of different approaches could be used. In order to limit the discussion to a realistic time frame and to my own experience, I chose to compare the BS/PharmD curriculum in which I was enrolled in 1969 to the entry level PharmD of 1989. One could have chosen to compare Bachelor Degree programs or PharmD programs. However, in discussing the clinical curriculum and its evolution, I chose to consider the curriculum evolution in terms of the progress made in the entry level PharmD program.

In 1969, the American Council on Pharmaceutical Education (ACPE) did not have guidelines for accreditation of an entry level PharmD Degree. The ACPE guidelines were for the accreditation of the Bachelor of Science in Pharmacy Degree. It was not until 1974 that the ACPE developed guidelines for accreditation that included clinical education. ACPE's new accreditation guidelines in 1974 required clinical clerkships for the first time. These standards called for separate accreditation for the Bachelor of Science Degree and the Doctor of Pharmacy Degree programs. However, one of the similarities in the two guidelines was that each had to include clinical sciences and practice experience gained through clerkships and externships in order to meet accreditation standards. Then, in 1975, the American Council on Pharmaceutical Education published accreditation guidelines for the Doctor of Pharmacy curriculum. These guidelines specified that the Doctor of Pharmacy Degree was a clinical education program.

As the clinical curriculum has progressed over the past twenty years, we have seen the development of new clinical courses, an improvement in the evaluation of teaching, a refinement of the ACPE evaluation process which includes a clinician on each site team. ACPE site teams have become more specific in their approach to their evaluation of programs looking for specific areas within clinical education, such as an emphasis on communication skills, drug literature evaluation and a variety of clinical experiences beyond just the four hundred hours that were originally required in 1974 for a BS Program. The changes in the ACPE standards and guidelines have indeed moved forward with the evolution of the clinical curriculum.

Curricular Changes

Suffice it to say the curriculum has changed dramatically in the past twenty years. These changes can be noted in the basic sciences, administrative sciences and clinical sciences. All three areas have been in a state of growth and change during the past twenty years. The 1969 curriculums were characterized by an emphasis on the biochemical sciences, specifically medicinal chemistry, inorganic medicinal chemistry, basic pharmacology, physical pharmacy, pharmacognosy, pharmaceutics, dispensing, physiology and microbiology. There was very little, if any, emphasis placed on topics such as pathology, chemotherapy, biostatistics, therapeutics, pharmacokinetics, or nutrition. Also these curriculums were heavily laden with laboratories which took a tremendous amount of time and manpower. We saw the first courses in biopharmaceutics during the late 60's, but few had a clinical emphasis.

As schools of pharmacy began to experiment with clinical curriculums and to realize the need for a more clinical emphasis, there had to be changes in the curriculum in order to find space for the new clinical programs. Even with adding a year to the Bachelor of Science Degree to make it a four year entry level PharmD Degree, there was not enough time within the traditional curriculum to present the material that had been presented historically, as well as the new clinically relevant matrial. The logical areas to decrease were the chemistry and pharmacognosy areas and the laboratories in the basic sciences. While all faculty did not agree with this approach, these are the areas that were reduced to make way for clinical education.

The following are the majority of the changes that have occurred in the pharmacy curriculum in the past twenty years:

1. A decrease, or in some cases elimination, of most laboratories from the pharmacy curriculum.

2. A shift away from an emphasis on the chemical sciences with a product orientation to the biological sciences with a patient orientation.

3. A greater emphasis on general education in the pre-pharmacy curriculum.

4. A focus on counseling and communication skills, both written and verbal.

5. A recognition of the need to be able to apply the basic sciences to the clinical sciences.

6. A shift to include more case studies and relevant materials to practice in both the clinical and the basic science courses. There are courses where basic science material must be presented and not necessarily with a relevance to practice, but to provide a base line of knowledge as well.

7. The development of tracking programs with emphasis on specific areas of pharmacy practice, *i.e.*, community pharmacy, hospital pharmacy, industry, clinical and/or graduate education. While tracking programs have not received universal approval from the academic community, they have become a major component of many of the curriculums of colleges in pharmacy. In some cases they have been tried and discarded and in other cases they have been modified to meet current student needs. These programs have been developed in both BS and PharmD programs.

8. An increased emphasis on specific therapeutic areas, such as geriatrics, pediatrics, psychiatry, cardiology, etc. Indeed, in 1969 you would be hard pressed to find a

Table 1. First professional year

Course Title	1969	BS	1989	PharmD
	Quarter hour credits			
Pharmacognosy (Natural drug products)	7	(6–3)	0	
Quantitative Analysis	6	(3–8)	0	
Accounting	2	(1–2)	0	
Organic Chemistry	5	(3–4)	0	
Biochemistry	5	(3–4)	8	(6–8)
Organic Medicinal Chemistry	0		10	(10–0)
Pharmacy Mathematics	3	(3–0)	2	(2–0)
Physical Pharmacy	4	(3–4)	4	(4–0)
Orientation in Pharmacy	0		2	(2–0)
Behavioral Sciences & Pharmacy Practice (Communications Skills)	0		3	(3–0)
Anatomy	0		2	(2–2)
Physiology	0		7	(7–0)
Pharmaceutical Technology	8	(6–8)	10	(8–8)
Introduction to Pharmacy Law	0		2	(2–0)
Health Care Administration	0		2	(2–0)
Total hours	43	(31–33)	50	(50–20)

Notes:
1. 1966–67 BS Curriculum.
2. The laboratory hours per week were reduced from 31 hours to 20 hours.
3. The courses eliminated from the curriculum include: pharmacognosy (natural drug products), accounting, quantitative analysis, and organic chemistry.
4. Courses not included in the first year curriculum in 1969 include: antomy, physiology, law, health care administration, communication skills and medicinal chemistry.
5. Refer to Table II for courses which were in the BS curriculum but not in the first professional year.
6. There are some changes between the two curriculums in course content that cannot be denoted by credit hours or course names.
7. Note that there is a significant increase in the quarter hour credits from the BS program to the PharmD program (43–50).

    course in therapeutics in any of the BS programs. In 1989 it is a standard component of, not only PharmD programs, but also BS programs as well.

9. The availability of elective clerkships have increased in the past five years in the area of research and instrumentation to stimulate pharmacy students' interest in postgraduate education and research. This is an area that needs to be developed more fully if we are to have basic scientists with pharmacy backgrounds in the future.

10. The development of a cadre or adjunct, part-time and volunteer faculty who provide a significant amount of our clinical education.

11. Clinical curriculums today are designed to prepare the student to select drug therapy regimens versus just product recognition. This not only reflects a change in philosophy, but a change in the student's knowledge base. Today, the student is encouraged to participate as a member of the health care team and to promote rational drug therapy. In 1969, the emphasis was on recognizing incompatibilities, compounding, and drug dispensing without the patient counseling and the provision of drug information to the physician. Therapeutic substitution was not encouraged or discussed in pharmacy education in 1969.

12. Curriculums today are trying to focus more on the future rather than limiting their outcomes to the present. The curriculums of 1969 were attempting to do this,

but it was not until the 1980s, in the author's opinion, that the emphasis has been placed on educating for the future.

13. A focus on patient assessment skills.

14. A major shift in emphasis in the professional practice component of the curriculum from the dispensing and externship experiments in 1969 to require clerkships and rotations in specific practice areas in 1989 in both BS and PharmD programs.

15. Outcome assessment requirements related to the curriculum are now being implemented by ACPE. In 1969 the term was not utilized in most circles and most definitely not in pharmacy education circles. Accountability is an issue which we must address today in higher education.

16. Educators are beginning to realize that we need to focus on the ability of the student to synthesize information rather than memorization for examinations. We have just scratched the surface in this area.

17. New courses in biotechnology are beginning to appear in curriculums as well as requirements in computer skills.

Table II. Second professional year

	Quarter hour credits			
Course Title	1969	BS	1989	PharmD
Analyatical Pharmaceutical Chemistry	4	(3–4)	0	
Pharmacognosy (Natural Drug Products)	3	(3–0)	0	
Pathophysiology	0		9	(9–0)
Microbiology	4	(3–2)	5	(4–4)
Physiology	8	(6–4)	0	
Medicinal Chemistry	8	(6–4)	0	
Biochemistry	3	(2–3)	0	
Pharmaceutical Technology	3	(3–0)	0	
Dispensing Pharmacy	8	(6–8)	2	(1–3)
Parenteral Medications	0		3	(2–2)
Pharmacy Pharmacology	0		9	(8–3)
Professional Practice Management	0		6	(6–0)
Drug Information Resources and Literature Retrieval & Evaluation	0		6	(4–4)
Bioharmaceutics	0		3	(3–0)
Biostatistics	0		3	(3–0)
Nonprescription Drugs	0		3	(3–0)
Chemical Toxicology	3	(3–0)	0	
Clinical Toxicology	0		3	(3–0)
Pharmacokinetics	0		3	(3–0)
Elective	0		3	(varies)
Total hours	44	(36–25)	58	(51–16)

Notes:
1. 1967–68 BS curriculum.
2. The laboratory hours per week were reduced from 25 hours to 16 hours. Also, it should be noted that the types of laboratories are significantly different. There are four hours of laboratory devoted to Drug Information in the PharmD program.
3. The courses eliminated from the curriculum include: analytical pharmaceutical chemistry, pharmacognosy, chemical toxicology (in 1989 focused on clinical toxicology), and physiology, medicinal chemistry, biochemistry, and pharmaceutical technology were moved to the first professional year and in some cases reduced in terms of credit hours.
4. There was a significant reduction in the amount of dispensing, reduced from eight hours to two hours but an increase in microbiology from four to five hours.
5. New courses added include: pathophysiology, parenteral medications, management courses, drug information courses, biostatistics and pharmacokinetics.

Table III. Third professional year

Course title	Quarter hour credits			
	1969	BS	1989	PharmD
Pharmacetutical Economics	3	(3–0)	0	
Preventive Medicine	3	(3–0)	0	
Pharmacy Pharmacology	9	(8–3)	0	
Retail Pharmacy Management	3	(3–0)	0	
Dispensing Pharmacy	12	(9–9)	0	
Applied Pharmacokinetics	0		3	(2–2)
Patient Assessment	0		3	(2–2)
Pharmaceutical Jurisprudence	3	(3–0)	3	(3–0)
Therapeutics Modules	0		23	(23–0)
Renal (2), Pulmonary (2), Cardiovascular (3), Hematology (2), Infectious Disease (2), Nutrition (1), Gastroinstestinal (2), Pediatric (1), Endocrinology-Reproduction (2), Psychopharmacology (2), Rheumatology (1), Oncology (1), Neurology (1), and Gerontology (1)				
Community Pharmacy Externship	0		5	(1–12)
Institutional Pharmacy Externship	0		5	(1–12)
Introductory Clerkship	0		2	(0–8)
Electives	8	(varies)	12	(varies)
Total hours	41	(37–12)	56	(32–36)

Notes:
1. 1968–69 BS curriculum.
2. There is again a significant difference in the laboratory hours, however there is an increase in the PharmD program laboratory hours. The difference is the introduction of the excternship program. In 1969, there was not a practice component with the exception of the dispensing laboratory. Of the 36 hours of laboratory in the PharmD program, 34 of those hours are practice based.
3. Note the change in the courses offered as well as the increased number of hours of electives.
4. The emphasis on therapeutics in the PharmD program of 1989 is the single greatest change in the curriculum.

The five tables in this section compare a 1969 BS/Post BS PharmD to a 1989 entry-level PharmD curriculum. In order to draw comparisons that are realistic, the comparison was made from the Bachelor of Science curriculum in 1969 of the University of Tennessee in years one, two and three and the Post BS PharmD program of the University of Tennessee in 1969 to the entry level PharmD curriculum in 1989 of the University of Tennessee. There is a significant difference in these two curriculums. Specifically those changes are summarized in Table V. Glaring changes include:

1. The introduction of courses to the curriculum including: communication skills, chemotherapy, over-the-counter products, biostatistics, pharmacokinetics, nutrition, anatomy, and the administrative sciences.

2. Courses that had slight changes in them include biochemistry, pharmacology, medicinal chemistry, and physiology.

The area that saw the greatest change was in the area of professional practice. In the entry level PharmD degree of 1989 there are forty-five quarter hours of clerkship and rotation experience in the fourth year. In the fourth year of the 1969 PharmD curriculum there were ten hours of clerkships. This reflects a significant change in the curriculum. This is typical of most programs which one might compare.

Table IV. Fourth professional year

Course title	Quarter hour credits			
	Post-BS 1969	PharmD	1989	PharmD
Clinical Pharmacy I–IV (Therapeutics and Clerkships Combined)	20	(8–36)	0	
Pharmacutical Operations I–IV (Combination Clerkships and pharmacy practice)	20	(8–36)	0	
Literature Resources in the Health Sciences	4	(2–6)	0	
Biopharmaceutics	3	(3–0)	0	
Computer Techniques	3	(2–3)	0	
Advanced Hospital Pharmacy	4	(4–0)	0	
Seminar in Pharmaceutical Sciences	1	(1–0)	0	
Hospital Administration	2	(2–0)	0	
Clinical Clerkships—Required	0		20	(0–160)
Clinical Clerkships Elective	0		15	(0–120)
Clinical Clerkships/Externship-Elective	0		10	(0–80)
Total hours	61	(34–81)	45	(0–360)

Notes:
1. 1969–70 post-BS/PharmD curriculum.
2. The significant difference in these two curriculums is the clinical practice component and the lack of didactic course work in the 1989 PharmD program in the fourth year.
3. This was the second year of the post-BS/PharmD program of the University of Tennessee and the curriculum was changing to meet two needs that were identified by the students. There were 12 students in the 1969–70 post-BS/PharmD program and the program was four quarters in length.
4. Much of the above didactic course work has been moved to the first three years of the PharmD curriculum or has been eliminated.

Most schools have either eliminated their wet labortories or limited them to demonstration labs via videotape or closed circuit TV. There are elective courses in research design and instrumentation that have been added to curriculums to meet the needs of those students who have a focused interest on research and/or graduate education. These courses have been successful in attracting students. However, their efforts need to be redoubled in the future to attract pharmacy students to post graduate education.

We, as faculty, must continually strive to improve our communication with and evaluation of adjunct faculty, in order to continue to enhance clinical education. Training programs without these individuals who serve as adjunct volunteer faculty would be impossible.

Teaching Skills and Techniques

Our teaching skills and techniques have definitely improved over the past twenty years. We have integrated clinical application into the basic science courses, implemented learning objectives, strengthened the evaluation process of our teaching and faculty, and begun to utilize technology, *i.e.*, computers, audio visuals and other study aids, in our educational process. We have also become more cognizant of the need to refine our curriculums with input from students and alumni and have begun the process of looking at the outcomes assessment.

Table V. Summary of curriculum changes

Course title	Quarter hour credits		
	1966–70	1989–93	Change
Pharmacognosy	10(9–7)	0	− 10
Quantitative Analysis	6(3–8)	0	− 6
Accounting	2(1–2)	0	− 2
Organic Chemistry	5(3–4)	0	− 5
Biochemistry	8(5–8)	8(6–8)	0
Organic Medicinal Chemistry	8(6–4)	10(10–10)	+ 2
Pharmacy Mathematics	3(3–0)	2(2–0)	− 1
Orientation in Pharmacy	3(3–0)	2(2–0)	− 1
Communication Skills	0	3(3–0)	+ 3
Anatomy	0	2(2–2)	+ 2
Physiology	8(6–4)	7(7–0)	− 1
Pharmaceutical Technology	11(9–8)	10(8–8)	+ 2
Pharmacy Jurisprudence	5(5–0)	5(5–0)	0
Pharmacy Management	6(6–0)	8(8–0)	+ 2
Analytical Pharm. Chemistry	4(3–4)	0	− 4
Pathophysiology	0	9(9–0)	+ 9
Microbiology	4(3–2)	5(4–4)	+ 1
Dispensing Pharmacy	20(15–17)	2(1–3)	− 18
Parenteral Medications	0	3(2–2)	+ 3
Pharmacy Pharmacology	9(8–3)	9(8–3)	0
Drug Information Retrieval &	6(6–6)	6(4–4)	0
Biopharmaceutics	3(3–0)	0	− 3
Nonprescription Drugs	0	3(3–0)	0
Chemical Toxicology	3(3–0)	0	− 3
Clinical Toxicology	0	3(3–0)	0
Pharmacokinetics	0	6(6–0)	+ 6
Electives	8(var.)	15(var.)	+ 7
Preventive Medicine	3(3–0)	0	− 3
Patient Assessment	0	3(2–2)	+ 3
Therapeutics	0	3(2–2)	+ 3
Externships	0	10(2–24)	+10
Introductory Clerkship	0	2(0–8)	+ 2
Clinical Pharmacy I–IV	20(8–36)	0	− 20
Pharmacuetical Oper. I–IV	20(8–36)	0	− 20
Computer Techniques	3(2–3)	0	− 3
Advanced Hospital Pharmacy	4(4–0)	0	− 4
Clinical Clerkships	0	45(0–360)	+45
Seminar in Pharm. Sciences	1(1–0)	0	− 1
Hospital Administration	2(2–0)	0	− 2
Total hours	189(138–151)	209(133–432)	

Notes: The actual credit hours increased by 20 quarter hours credits and the actual basic science laboratory hours decreased from 70 in the BS program to 36 in the PharmD program.

However, we have just scratched the surface. We still have a tendency to teach from a pedagogical approach rather than an andragogical approach to education. We have slipped into using too many objective tests because of the need to save time. We need to improve our understanding of basic educational principles in order to enhance clinical education and indeed the entire educational process. If we are to continue to make the same amount of progress over the next twenty years that we have over the last twenty, then we, as professors and educators, will need to focus our attention on new educational techniques and continue to improve on those that we use today. We must focus attention on the quality of our teaching conducted by our faculty, both in the basic and clinical sciences. Implementation of staff development programs to teach the faculty how to teach, is critical to the long term success of pharmacy education.

How do you teach students to learn and to study? How do you stimulate students to become excited and enthused about the profession and indeed in learning itself? This is not a problem that pharmacy has alone, but is indicative of the entire educational system. We have made tremendous strides in the educational system within pharmacy, but need to continue to progress for the future.

Summary

Curriculum evolution, what progress have we made?—Tremendous strides! In twenty years we have changed the face of pharmacy education. During this short span of time we have changed the makeup of faculty, changed the curriculum, changed the focus of the curriculum from the basic sciences to the applied clinical sciences with a biological emphasis. In no other health profession has there been so great a change in such a short period of time. When one reviews and compares the curriculum of 1969 to that of 1989, it shows a tremendous degree of change and emphasis. This does not mean that the curriculums and programs of 1969 were bad or inadequate, it just means that we have met the changing needs and demands of the health care system in which we work.

In answer to the question—What progress have we made? Dramatic progress has been made, but more needs to be made for the future. The challenges which we will face in the future will be to continue to evolve the clinical education from which we have now begun to reap benefits. To rest on our laurels now, would be showing benign neglect to the profession and to the health and welfare of the public which we serve.

In the future we will need to place more emphasis on outcomes assessment, faculty development and evaluation, developing an andragogical approach to education and to the development of our graduate education and post graduate education programs which will focus on the needs of the future.

Contemporary Pharmacy Education

Components of Pharmacy Education

Pharmacy education is divided into three major stages.

1. Prepharmacy education, which requires two years as a minimum and may be taken at a junior college, community college, four-year college, or a university (time may be reduced by taking an accelerated load, although this is not necessarily recommended).

2. Professional pharmacy education, which takes either three years (B.S. degree) or four years (Pharm.D. degree) and must be taken at one of the 74 schools or colleges of pharmacy in the United States.

3. Postghraduate education, which is comprised of either graduate education leading to a M.S., M.B.A., or Ph.D.; a residency or fellowship program; or professional continuing pharmaceutical education.

Degrees Offered

There are two professional pharmacy degrees offered in pharmacy college:

1. The Bachelor of Science in Pharmacy—B.S.
2. The Doctor of Pharmacy—Pharm.D.

The graduate degrees offered in the pharmaceutical sciences include the following:

1. Master of Science—M.S.
2. Doctor of Philosophy—Ph.D.

Fifty-four pharmacy colleges have graduate programs. The graduate programs in the pharmaceutical sciences at the master's level are usually offered in areas of medicinal chemistry, pharmaceutics, pharmacy administration, pharmacology, toxicology pharmacokinetics, and nuclear pharmacy. This list is not all-inclusive. The Ph.D. degree is also offered in these areas in many colleges as well. There are a number of colleges of pharmacy that offer a joint Pharm.D./Ph.D. program. To enter these programs students must have a previously earned B.S. degree in an area other than pharmacy and must take all of their electives in the graduate school.

Another very popular combined graduate program is the joint B.S./M.B.A. or Pharm.D./M.B.A. These programs are offered in a number of colleges of pharmacy in conjunction with a school of business. Students with the joint degree are very attractive to the pharmaceutical industry as well as the chain drugstore industry.

Prepharmacy Curriculum

Course	Minimal Quarter Hours	Minimal Hours
General Chemistry	12	8
Organic Chemistry	12	9
General Biology/Zoology	12	8
Physics	12	8
English Composition	9	6
Speech	3	3
Accounting	3	3
Fundamentals of Calculus	3	3
Social Science Electives	9	6
(Psychology, Sociology, Economics, Anthropology, Political Science, etc.)	9	6
Humanities Electives (Literature, Language, History, Philosophy, etc.)	9	6
General Electives	15	7
TOTAL	99	66

Note: One year of American History (high school or college level) is required for graduation from the University of Tennessee.

For information on graduate education programs, joint undergraduate professional and graduate degree programs, contact the school or college of pharmacy that you are considering to determine the graduate degree programs that are available.

Prepharmacy Requirements

Pharmacy collegs require two years of prepharmacy for entrance into the professional curriculum. Students with a minimum of two years of college are eligible for entrance into pharmacy colleges as long as the basic prepharmacy requirements are met. The prepharmacy requirements for students applying to colleges of pharmacy are a minimum of two years. This minimum might be either sixty semester hours or ninety quarter hours, depending upon the particular program. The following minimum requirements for admission have been established by the University of Tennessee College of Pharmacy, They provide an idea of what one program's requirements are like: Completion of 59 semester hours of required prepharmacy courses, and 7 semester hours of elective courses, for a total of 66 semester hours.

Minimum keyboard skills of 40 words per minute will be required of students prior to the third year of the professional curriculum. A formal course in keyboard skills is not offered by the College of Pharmacy.

All colleges of pharmacy will vary to some degree in their requirements; the major differences will be in the number of required hours in physics, organic chemistry, and mathematics students. should contact each institution to which they are applying for specific information about that institution's requirements.

Professional Curriculum

The professional curriculum in colleges of pharmacy has changed dramatically over the past twenty years. Until 1948, colleges of pharmacy required a total of four years of education; however, today the minimum requirement is five years, with two years generally for completing the prepharmacy requirements and three years in the professional curriculum. Colleges of pharmacy that offer a bachelor's degree offer three years of professional curriculum, whereas those that offer the Pharm.D. degree as the entry-level degree offer four years.

The basic pharmacy curriculum is comprised of basic science and clinical science courses. The following are examples of two curricula, one a B.S curriculum (The University of Mississippi) and the other a Pharm.D. curriculum (The University of Tennessee). These two curricula will provide you with an idea of the intensity and content of the pharmacy curriculum.

Bachelor of Science Curriculum (University of Mississippi)
First Professional Year

Prepharmacy Program (two years)
Minimum Total: 34 Semester Hours

	Clock Hours per Week		Semester Hours	
Courses	Lecture	Laboratory	First	Second
Biological Sciences 160, 161, 162, 163			8	
Chemistry 105, 106	3, 3		3	3
Chemistry 115, 116		3, 3	1	1
English 101, 102[1]	3, 3		3	3
Mathematics 121, 123[2]	3, 3		3	3
Electives[3]	6		6	

Second Professional Year

Minimum Total: 34 Semester Hours

	Clock Hours per Week		Semester Hours	
Courses	Lecture	Laboratory	First	Second
Chemistry 221, 222	3, 3		3	3
Chemistry 225, 226		3, 3	1	1
Biological Sciences 33	2	4	4	
Physics 213, 214	3, 3		3	3
Physics 223, 224		2, 2	1	1
Electives[3]			15	

Professional Program (Three Years) B.S. First Professional Year

Minimum Total: 30 Semester Hours

	Clock Hours per Week		Semester Hours	
Courses	Lecture	Laboratory	First	Second
Medicinal Chemistry, 311	3		3	
Pharmaceutics 345, 346	3, 2	3, 3	4	3
Pharmacology 361, 362	3, 3	3, 3	4	4
Pharmacology 373	3			3
Health Care Administration 381, 382	3, 3		3	3
Medicinal Chemistry 312	2	3	3	

Second Professional Year

Minimum Total: 30 Semester Hours

	Clock-Hours per Week		Semester Hours	
Courses	Lecture	Laboratory	First	Second
Medicinal Chemistry 403, 404	3, 3		3	3
Pharmaceutics 445	3	3	4	
Clinical Pharmacy Practice 448	3			3
Clinical Pharmacy Practice 449		3		1
Pharmacognosy 425, 426	4, 3	3	4	4
Pharmacology 563, 564	3, 4	3	4	4
Health Care Administration 480	2		2	

Third Professional Year

Minimum Total: 29 Semester Hours

	Clock-Hours per Week		Semester Hours	
Courses	Lecture	Laboratory	First	Second
Pharmaceutics 546	3	3	4	
Pharmaceutics 548	2		2	
Clinical Pharmacy Practice 552, 353	6, 6		6, 6	
Health Care Administration 581	2		2	
Health Care Administration 580	2		2	
Health Care Administration 583	4		4	
Electives	4		4	

Doctor of Pharmacy Curriculum (University of Tennessee)

First Professional Year

Fall Semester

ANAT 121	Anatomy	3(202)
BIOC 111	Biochemistry	5(4–2)
MEDC 112	Medicinal Chemistry	3(3–0)
HSAD 132	Pharmacy and the Health Care Environment	2(1–2)
PHAC 111	Physical Pharmacy and Math	4(4–0)
Total		17(15–6)

Spring Semester

MEDC 122	Medicinal Chemistry II	3(3–0)
PHYS 121	Physiology	5(4–1)
PHAC 123	Pharmaceutical Technology	5(4–4)
MICR 211	Microbiology and Immunology	4(3–2)
HSAD 121	Counseling and Communication	2(1–3)
	Elective (optional)	varies
Total		19+(16+ – 10+)

Second Professional Year

Fall Semester

PHAR 211	Pharmacology I	4(3–2)
PHAC 212	Parenterals	2(1–2)
PHAC 221	Biopharmaceutics	2(2–0)
CLPH 231	Nonprescription Drugs	3(3–0)
HSAD 211	Professional Practice Management	3(3–0)
BIOE 221	Biostatistics	2(2–0)
	Elective	2(varies)
Total		18(13+ – 8+)

Spring Semester

MICR 211	Microbiology & Immunology	4(3–2)
MEDC 211	Pathophysiology I	2(2–0)
PHAR 221	Pharmacology II	3(3–0)
CLPH 221	Drug Information and Literature Evaluation	3(2–2)
PHAC 233	Pharmacokinetics	3(2–2)
CLPH 315	Patient Assessment	2(1–2)
	Elective	2(varies)
Total		19(13+ – 8+)

Third Professional Year

Fall Semester

CLPH 316	Therapeutics I	6(5–2)
CKPH 317	Therapeutics II	6(5–2)
CLPH 315	Patient Assessment	2(1–1)
CKPH 324	Clinical Pharmacokinetics	1(1–2)
HSAD 322	Pharmacy Correlation Conference	1(1–0)
	Elective	2(varies)
Total		19(13+ – 8+)

Spring Semester

CLPH 318	Therapeutics III	5(4–2)
CLPH 319	Therapeutics IV	5(4–2)
HSAD 321	Pharmaceutical Jurisprudence	2(2–0)
CKPH 338	Introductory Clerkship	1(0–4)
HSAD 310	Community Externship	3(0–10)
HSAD 320	Institutional Externship	3(0–10)
	Elective	2(varies)
Total		21(8+ – 28+)

As you will note from the above curriculum, there is a significant amount of basic science coursework, including biochemistry, pathology, anatomy, physiology, medical microbiology, as well as pharmaceutical chemistry and pharmacology. Other courses, such as nonprescription products, communication skills, toxicology, and drug literature evaluation, are also included in many curricula.

The clinical science area of the curriculum deals with professional practice. The curriculum of the final professional year is heavily oriented toward pharmacy practice. Students do clerkships, where they learn to apply what they know in actual pharmacy practice. At clerkship sites, students train under registered pharmacists alongside medical and nursing students in a "health care team" approach. Students can obtain clerkship experience in such settings as community pharmacies, drug information centers, adult medical units, pediatric units, psychiatric units, ambulatory clinics, nursing homes,

Fourth Professional Year

Fall Semester

CLPH 411	Clinical Clerkship I	3(0–10)
CLPH 412	Clinical Clerkship II	3(0–10)
CLPH 413	Clinical Clerkship III	3(0–10)
CLPH 414	Clinical Clerkship IV	3(0–10)
Clerkship (elective)		3(0–10)
Total		15(0–50)

Spring Semester

Clerkship (elective)	3(0–10)
Clerkship (elective)	3(0–10)
Clerkship or externship (elective)	3(0–10)
Clerkship or externship (elective)	3(0–10)
Total	12(0–40)

pharmaceutical manufacturing firms, and nuclear pharmacies. At these sites, students provide a variety of services to patients, including dispensing medications, educating patients about their drug therapy, conducting medication history interviews, and monitoring drug therapy. They also provide drug information to other health care professionals and serve as consultants when decisions are made on drug therapy.

The Pharm. D. curriculums require a minimum of 1,500 hours of professional practice experience. The University of Tennessee requires 1,960 hours of externship/clerkship. These hours are obtained by completing 12 one-month experiences of 160 hours per month. The amount of clinical experience required in a B.S. program is a minimum of 400 hours of clerkship, versus 1,500 hours in Pharm.D. programs. Both degrees are considered entry-level degrees for the profession of pharmacy. The trend over the past several years has been the development of more Pharm.D. programs in colleges of pharmacy. For information on each pharmacy college's curriculum you should write to the dean's office of the college in which you are interested. The addresses of the accredited colleges of pharmacy in the United States appear later in this chapter.

Pharmacy is an ever-changing profession, as are the educational programs of the pharmacy colleges. Most major colleges, as well as community colleges, have health profession advisors. Students currently enrolled in an institution that has no college of pharmacy should seek advice from a health professions advisor and particularly from the individual who serves as the prepharmacy advisor.

Choosing a Pharmacy Program

What is the choice that you as a prospective pharmacy student should make in selecting your pharmacy degree program? Should you enter a B.S. or a Pharm.D. program? Sara Martin in a recent issue of the *Pharmacy Student* suggested the following:

1. Ask yourself what you want. It's hard to know what you'll be doing even a year after graduation, but ask yourself: Will the opportunities that are available with a B.S. satisfy me in five to ten years? What kind of practice interests me? Will it require a Pharm.D.?

2. Ask your local pharmacists what they think, and what their experiences have been.

3. Ask your advisors what they recommend.

4. Research your interests. Keep up to date with the changes in the profession of pharmacy.[1]

How does the Doctor of Pharmacy curriculum differ from the Bachelor of Science curriculum?

The doctor of pharmacy (Pharm.D.) curriculum emphasizes a more patient-oriented course of study than does the B.S. curriculum. This curriculum offers advanced courses in areas such as therapeutics, pathophysiology, biostatistics, and pharmacokinetics, which may not be required in the typical B.S. program. The Pharm.D. curriculum also provides an additional year of clinical (practice experience) clerkships that are primarily devoted to patient assessment and counseling, and drug therapy monitoring as well as traditional dispensing roles. Pharm.D. programs require a minimum of 1,500 hours of practice, while B.S. programs require a minimum of 400 hours.

Can students obtain a B.S. degree and then return for a Pharm.D. degree?

Yes, there are many schools that offer a postbaccalaureate Pharm.D. degree; however, their class size is very small, and admission is competitive. Additionally, these programs are normally two calendar years in length, which means that it will take seven years to get the Pharm.D. degree rather than six years, as in an entry-level program.

What are the job opportunities for a Doctor of Pharmacy graduate?

Pharm.D.s are qualified to do **all** jobs performed by B.S. graduates. Moreover, the Pharm.D. is qualified for highly specialized fields. At the 24th Annual meeting of the American Society of Hospital Pharmacists, December 1989, over 60 percent of the jobs posted in the Placement Service showed preference to Pharm.D. graduates over B.S. graduates.

Can the Pharm.D. candidates specialize in a chosen area?

Most Pharm.D. programs have opportunities for students to take electives and to develop areas of emphasis such as: pharmacokinetics, metabolic support, nuclear pharmacy, pediatrics, drug information, mental health, geriatrics, infectious disease, home health care, community pharmacy, industrial pharmacy, and other.

Are postdoctoral residencies available?

Upon completion of the doctor of pharmacy degree, there are a number of residency options available to graduates. The various residency programs include general hospital

---

[1]The following questions and answers should give you more of the information you need to make the decision that is right for you.

pharmacy residencies, specialty residencies, clinical residencies, and fellowships. A general residency or clinical residency is normally completed prior to the fellowship. Residencies are accredited by the American Society of Hospital Pharmacists (ASHP) at the present time, and a number of new residency programs are being developed in community and other ambulatory care settings. Residency descriptions and information can be obtained from the American Society of Hospital Pharmacists. Residency programs in the community are detailed in further information available from the American Pharmaceutical Association and American College of Apothecaries.

How will future roles of pharmacists differ from present roles?

The future financing and organization of health care is changing very rapidly. As the health care system changes, so do the professions within the system. New laws in several states permit pharmacists to become actively involved in the prescribing of medications. We will see a continous evolution of the pharmacists's role from being a dispenser of medications to that of a health practitioner with greater control over the selection, dispensing, and administration of medicines.

Do the anticipated changes in roles for the future necessitate a change in education?

Education will meet the future needs of the pharmacy practitioner. Greater emphasis will be placed on high technology, wellness care, self-care computer applications, and other innovations in order to prepare pharmacists for new responsibilities. Doctor of pharmacy degree programs have evolved over the years in response to changing demands for specialized instruction and training.

What factors should be considered in selecting a program for your professional pharmacy education?

Choosing a college or school of pharmacy is an extremely important and often difficult decision. Many factors should be evaluated, but the primary goal is to select the program that offers the highest quality of education and level of service. The institution's commitment to academic excellence and genuine concern for the student's needs are also important selection criteria. The location and setting, specifically the types and varieties of clinical and training facilities, are important factors.

Financial Aid for Pharmacy Students

There is a variety of financial aid available for study in pharmacy programs. You may, for instance, be eligible for one or more of the following federal aid programs:

Pell Grants
College Work Study
Perkins Loans (formerly National Defense Student Loans)
Supplemental Educational Opportunity Grants (SEOG)

Stafford Student Loans (formerly Guaranteed Student Loans)
Health Professional Student Loans (HPSL)
Health Education Assistance Loans (HEAL)
Veterans Benefits
Supplemental Loans for Students (SLS)

For more information about eligibility for these programs, and how you can apply, write to the United States Department of Education or call the Federal Student Aid Information Center at 1–800–333–INFO.

In addition to federal programs, many states offer need-based and/or merit scholarships to students who attend state-supported institutions.

Each college and university also has its own financial aid program, and may offer loans, grants, and scholarships. You should request financial aid information from each of the pharmacy programs to which you may apply.

Many private foundations and organizations also have scholarship programs. Most libraries will have directories listing foundation and other private grants to individuals. Libraries will also carry reference volumes that describe in detail all forms and sources of financial aid for undergraduate and graduate study.

Postgraduate Education: Residencies and Fellowships

In 1953 the American Society of Hospital Pharmacists (ASHP) began the accreditation of postgraduate training programs in hospital pharmacy. There programs were called hospital pharmacy residencies. During the past twenty years, the proliferation of residency programs has been dramatic. The ASHP is the accrediting body for hospital pharmacy residencies as well as specialty residencies. There are 153 accredited residency programs in the United States, as well as other nonaccredited fellowship programs. The number is growing every year.

About pharmacy residencies*
What is a pharmacy residency?

A pharmacy residency is an organized, directed postgraduate learning experience in a defined area of pharmacy practice.

What types of pharmacy residencies are there?

The most common type is the residency in hospital pharmacy practice, which is conducted in a hospital under the preceptorship of the director of the pharmacy department. The objective of residency training in hospital pharmacy practice is to develop competent practitioners who are able to provide a broad scope of pharmaceutical services (clinical services, informational services, drug distribution serivces, product formulation,

*From the ASHP publication *What Is a Pharmacy Residency*. Reprinted with permission of the American Society of Hospital Pharmacists.

quality control, supportive administrative services, etc.). Training typically involves structured rotations within the pharmacy department as well as other departments in the hospital, conferences and seminars, research projects, and related activities. Many residencies also provide for limited experience in pharmacies in other hospitals or other organized health care settings.

A second type is the residency of clinical pharmacy practice, which emphasizes the provision of clinical pharmacy services in organized health care settings to a wide variety of patients. Although most of the resident's training takes place in a hospital, less emphasis is placed on the overall operation of a hospital pharmacy than is the case in the residency in a hospital pharamcy as described above. Most residencies in clinical pharmacy are available only to those who have completed the Pharm.D. degree.

Specialized pharmacy residencies are a third category. Such residencies concentrate exclusively on one narrow area of pharmacy practice. Examples include psychiatric pharmacy practice, nuclear pharmacy, and nutrition support services.

What is meant by an "accredited" residency?

The accrediting body for the types of residencies described above is the American Society of Hospital Pharmacists. The society grants accreditation to institutions that meet certain standards of practice and which have demonstrated that they can provide a good training program. Accreditation of a pharmacy residency program by the society provides a certain assurance to prospective residents that the program has met these basic requirements and is therefore an acceptable site for postgraduate training in pharmacy practice.

What length of time is required to complete a pharmacy residency?

A minimum of two thousand hours of training extending over a minimum of fifty weeks is required in an ASHP-accredited residency program; this is the equivalent of one normal work year. Some residency programs are offered only in conjunction with an advanced degree (either an M.S. or a Pharm.D. degree) in a college of pharmacy or graduate school. Such programs are commonly referred to an "affiliated" residencies and generally require two years for completion. Residents in some affiliated programs pursue the residency on a part-time basis so there will be adequate time for course work, thesis research, and the other degree requirements. Many affiliated programs, however, allow the residency to be taken either before or after the postgraduate academic course work. Other residency programs ("nonaffiliated" residencies) are offered independently of an advanced degree and typically require one year of full-time work for completion. An applicant who already holds an advanced degree would normally choose one of these programs if he or she is interested in pursuing residency training.

Do residents earn a salary?

All accredited residency programs provide the resident with a stipend, although the amount varies from program to program, depending on such factors as the number of actual residency training hours per year, the value of any fringe benefits provided, and geographic location (cost of living). Cash stipends generally are inadequate to cover living costs for a resident having significant family support responsibilities. Furthermore, a residency, whether affiliated or nonaffiliated, requires a full-time commitment on the part of the resident and usually does not permit part-time employment to supplement income. For these reasons, applicants with family support obligations should have financial resources in addition to the residency stipend upon which they can rely during the residency training period.

Who should consider taking an accredited pharmacy residency?

Any pharmacist or pharmacy student whose career objectives center around institutional or clinical pharmacy practice should give serious consideration to residency training. Because of the concentrated nature of the training in a residency program, an individual may develop competence in a broader scope of pharmacy practice in a one- or two- year residency program than might be expected from several years as a staff pharmacist with a fixed assignment. Many "positions available" listings in the ASHP Personnel Placement Service specify completion of an accredited residency as an employment prerequisite.

What are the requirements for admission to an accredited pharmacy residency?

An applicant must be a graduate of an ACPE-accredited college of pharmacy (or must have graduated prior to the beginning date of the residency) and should have demonstrated an interest in and aptitude for advanced training in pharmacy. Some residencies require that the applicant be licensed to practice before entering the program, although others will accept applicants who have some limited internship obligation remaining for completion of state board licensure requirements. In the case of an affiliated residency program, the applicant must satisfy the requirements of the college of pharmacy or graduate school for admission to the advanced degree program, in addition to the requirements established by the institution in which the residency is offered. Residents in ASHP-accredited programs should be members of the American Society of Hospital Pharmacists.

Students with B.S. or Pharm.D. degrees who are applying for postgraduate residency and/or fellowship programs should write to the American Society of Hospital Pharmacists residency Matching Program, 4630 Montgomery Avenue, Bethesda, Maryland 20814. ASHP can provide a list of accredited residencies upon request.

United States Colleges and Schools of Pharmacy

ALABAMA
School of Pharmacy
Auburn University
Alabama 36849-5501
(205) 844-4740

School of Pharmacy
Samford University
800 Lakeshore Drive
Birmingham, Alabama 35229
(205) 870-2820

ARIZONA
College of Pharmacy
The University of Arizona
Tucson, Arizona 85721
(602) 626-1427

ARKANSAS
College of Pharmacy
University of Arkansas for Medical
    Sciences
4301 West Markham - Slot 522
Little Rock, Arkansas 72205-7122
(501) 686-5557

CALIFORNIA
School of Pharmacy
University of California
San Francisco, California 94143-0446
(415) 476-1225

School of Pharmacy
University of the Pacific
3601 Pacific Avenue
Stockton, California 95211
(209) 946-2561

School of Pharmacy
University of Southern California
1985 Zonal Avenue
Los Angeles, California 90033-1086
(213) 224-7501

COLORADO
School of Pharmacy
University of Colorado
Box 297
Boulder, Colorado 80309-0297
(303) 492-6278

CONNECTICUT
School of Pharmacy
The University of Connecticut
Box U-92 372 Fairfield Road
Storrs, Connecticut 06269-2092
(203) 486-2129

DISTRICT OF COLUMBIA
College of Pharmacy and Pharmacal
    Sciences
Howard University
2300 4th Street, N.W.
Washington, DC 20059
(202) 636-6530

FLORIDA
College of Pharmacy and
    Pharmaceutical Sciences
Florida Agricultural and Mechanical
    University
P.O. Box 367
Tallahassee, Florida 32307
(904) 599-3578

Southeastern College of Pharmaceutical
    Sciences
1750 N.E. 168th Street
N. Miama Beach, Florida 33162-3097
(305) 949-4000

College of Pharmacy
University of Florida
Box J-484
Health Science Center
Gainesville, Florida 32610
(904) 392-3405

GEORGIA
Southern School of Pharmacy
Mercer University
345 Boulevard, N.E.
Atlanta, Georgia 30312
(404) 653-8800

College of Pharmacy
The University of Georgia
Athens, Georgia 30602
(404) 542-1911

IDAHO
College of Pharmacy
Idaho State University
Pocatello, Idaho 83209-0009
(208) 236-2175

ILLINOIS
College of Pharmacy
University of Illinois at Chicago
833 South Wood St., Box 6998
M/C 874
Chicago, Illinois 60680-6998
(312) 996-7240

INDIANA
College of Pharmacy
Butler University
46th & Sunset Avenue
Indianapolis, Indiana 46208
(317) 283-9322

School of Pharmacy and Pharmacal
   Sciences
Purdue University
West Lafayette, Indiana 47907-0708
(317) 494-1357

IOWA
College of Pharmacy
Drake University
28th & Forest
Des Moines, Iowa 50311
(515) 271-2172

College of Pharmacy
The University of Iowa
Iowa City, Iowa 52242
(319) 335-8794

KANSAS
School of Pharmacy
University of Kansas
2056 Malott
Lawrence, Kansas 66045-2500
(913) 864-3591

KENTUCKY
College of Pharmacy
University of Kentucky
Rose Street - Pharmacy Building
Lexington, Kentucky 40536-0082
(606) 257-2738

LOUISIANA
School of Pharmacy
Northest Louisiana University
700 University Avenue
Monroe, Louisiana 71209-0470
(318) 342-2180

College of Pharmacy
Xavier University of Louisiana
7325 Palmetto Street
New Orleans, Louisiana 70125
(504) 483-7424

MARYLAND
School of Pharmacy
University of Maryland
20 North Pine Street
Baltimore, Maryland 21201-1180
(301) 328-7650

MASSACHUSETTS
Massachusetts College of Pharmacy and
   Allied Health Services
179 Longwood Avenue
Boston, Massachusetts 02115
(617) 732-2800

College of Pharmacy and Allied Health
   Professions
Northeastern University
360 Huntington Avenue
Boston, Massachusetts 02115
(617) 437-3321

MICHIGAN
School of Pharmacy
Ferris State University
901 South State Street
Big Rapids, Michigan 49307
(616) 592-2254

College of Pharmacy
The University of Michigan
Ann Arbor, Michigan 48109-1065
(313) 764-7312

College of Pharmacy and Allied Health
   Professions
Wayne State University
139 Shapero Hall
Detroit, Michigan 48202-3489
(313) 577-1716

MINNESOTA
College of Pharmacy
University of Minnesota
5-130 Health Sciences Unit F
308 Harvard Street, S.E.
Minneapolis, Minnesota 55455-0343
(612) 624-1900

MISSISSIPPI
School of Pharmacy
The University of Mississippi
University, Mississippi 38677-9814
(601) 232-7265

MISSOURI
St. Louis College of Pharmacy
4588 Parkview Place
St. Louis, Missouri 63110-1088
(314) 367-8700

School of Pharmacy
University of Missouri - Kansas City
5005 Rockhill Road
Kansas City, Missouri 64110
(816) 276-1607

MONTANA
School of Pharmacy and Allied Health
   Sciences
University of Montana
Missoula, Montana 59812
(406) 243-4621

NEBRASKA
School of Pharmacy and Allied Health
   Professions
Creighton University
California at 24th Street
Omaha, Nebraska 68178
(402) 280-2950

College of Pharmacy
University of Nebraska
42nd & Dewey Avenue
Omaha, Nebraska 68105-1065
(402) 559-4333

NEW JERSEY
College of Pharmacy
Rutgers University
The State University of New Jersey
Post Office Box 789
Piscataway, New Jersey 08855-0789
(201) 932-2666

NEW MEXICO
College of Pharmacy
University of New Mexico
Albuquerque, New Mexico 87131
(505) 277-2461

NEW YORK
Arnold & Marie Schwartz
College of Pharmacy and Health
   Sciences
Long Island University
75 DeKalb Ave. at University Plaza
Brooklyn, New York 11201
(718) 403-1060

College of Pharmacy and Allied Health
   Professions
St. John's University
Grand Central and Utopia Parkways
Jamaica, New York 11439
(718) 990-6275

School of Pharmacy
State University of New York at Buffalo
C126 Cooke-Hochstetter Complex
Buffalo, New York 14260
(716) 636-2823

Albany College of Pharmacy
Union University
106 New Scotland
Albany, New York 12208
(518) 445-7211

NORTH CAROLINA
School of Pharmacy
Campbell University
Post Office Box 1090
Buies Creek, North Carolina 27506
(919) 893-4111

School of Pharmacy
University of North Carolina
Beard Hall #7360
Chapel Hill, North Carolina
27599-7360
(919) 966-1121

NORTH DAKOTA
College of Pharmacy
North Dakota State University
Fargo, North Dakota 58105
(701) 237-7456

OHIO
College of Pharmacy
Ohio Northern University
Ada, Ohio 45810
(419) 772-2275

College of Pharmacy
The Ohio State University
500 West 12th Avenue
Columbus, Ohio 43210-1291
(614) 292-2266

College of Pharmacy
University of Cincinnati - Medical
    Center
Mail Location #4
Cincinnati, Ohio 45267
(513) 558-3784

College of Pharmacy
The University of Toledo
2801 West Bancroft Street
Toledo, Ohio 43606
(419) 537-2019

OKLAHOMA
School of Pharmacy
Southwestern Oklahoma State
    University
100 Campus Drive
Weatherford, Oklahoma 73096
(405) 774-3105

College of Pharmacy
University of Oklahoma
P.O. Box 26901
Oklahoma City, Oklahoma 73190-5040
(405) 271-6484

OREGON
College of Pharmacy
Oregon State University
Corvallis, Oregon 97331-3507
(503) 737-3424

PENNSYLVANIA
School of Pharmacy
Duquesne University
Pittsburgh, Pennsylvania 15282
(412) 434-6380

School of Pharmacy
Philadelphia College of Pharmacy and
    Science
Woodland Avenue at 43rd Street
Philadelphia, Pennsylvania 19104
(215) 596-8800

School of Pharmacy
Temple University
3307 North Broad Street
Philadelphia, Pennsylvania 19140
(215) 221-4990

School of Pharmacy
University of Pittsburgh
1103 Salk Hall
Pittsburgh, Pennsylvania 15261
(412) 648-8579

PUERTO RICO
College of Pharmacy
University of Puerto Rico
GPO Box 5067
San Juan, Puerto Rico 00936-5067
(809) 758-2525 (ext) 5400

RHODE ISLAND
College of Pharmacy
University of Rhode Island
Kingston, Rhode Island 02881-0809
(401) 792-2761

SOUTH CAROLINA
College of Pharmacy
Medical University of South Carolina
171 Ashley Avenue
Charleston, South Carolina
29425-2301
(803) 792-3115

College of Pharmacy
University of South Carolina
Columbia, South Carolina 29208
(803) 777-4151

SOUTH DAKOTA
College of Pharmacy
South Dakota State University
Box 2202C
Brookings, South Dakota 57007-0197
(605) 688-6197

TENNESSEE
College of Pharmacy
University of Tennessee
874 Union Avenue
Memphis, Tennessee 38163
(901) 528-6036

TEXAS

College of Pharmacy and Health
  Sciences
Texas Southern University
3100 Cleburne
Houston, Texas 77004
(713) 527-7164

College of Pharmacy
University of Houston
4800 Calhoun
Houston, Texas 77204-5511
(713) 749-4106

College of Pharmacy
University of Texas at Austin
Austin, Texas 78712-1074
(512) 471-1737

UTAH

College of Pharmacy
University of Utah
Salt Lake City, Utah 84112
(801) 581-6731

VIRGINIA

School of Pharmacy
Virginia Commonwealth University
MCV Campus - Box 581
410 North 12th Street
Richmond, Virginia 23298-0581
(804) 786-7346

WASHINGTON

School of Pharmacy
University of Washington
T-341 Health Science Center, SC-69
Seattle, Washington 98195
(206) 543-2030

College of Pharmacy
Washington State University
Pullman, Washington 99164-6510
(509) 335-8664

WEST VIRGINIA

School of Pharmacy
West Virginia University Health
  Sciences Center
Morgantown, West Virginia 26506
(304) 293-5101

WISCONSIN

School of Pharmacy
University of Wisconsin - Madison
425 North Charter Street
Madison, Wisconsin 53706
(608) 262-1416

WYOMING

School of Pharmacy
University of Wyoming
P. O. Box 3375
Laramie, Wyoming 82071-3375
(307) 766-6120

PART THREE

PHARMACY LICENSURE

Pharmacy Licensure

Intern Licensure

Upon registration in pharmacy college, students are eligible to file for internship licensure within the state in which they are enrolled. All states require internship hours (hours of practical experience in pharmacy practice under the tutelage of a pharmacy preceptor who is a licensed practitioner in the state in which the student is registered). The minimum number of required internship hours is 1,500. The majority of state boards of pharmacy require 1,500 hours and these hours may be obtained during the summer breaks between the professional years in the college of pharmacy or after graduation. Some state boards of pharmacy require that a minimum number of these hours be obtained after graduation. The current trend is away from this, so that students may take the state board of pharmacy examination upon graduation to become licensed. The boards of pharmacy may also give students credit for up to four hundred hours of internship credit obtained during the clinical curriculum of a college of pharmacy; some boards of pharmacy give more than four hundred hours. For specific information on how many hours of internship will be granted, and on the specific areas of practice that will be allowed for internship credit, the state board in question should be contacted. A listing of state boards of pharmacy follows later in this chapter.

Pharmacy Licensure Requirements

After graduation, students must take a theoretical and practical examination administered by a state board of pharmacy. The National Association of Boards of Pharmacy's standardized NABPLEX exam is administered by all state boards of pharmacy, with the exception of California and Louisiana. These two states make up their own licensure examinations. The NABPLEX is administered several times a year. Each state board adheres to a standardized set of dates for giving the exam. These dates can be obtained from each individual state board of pharmacy office.

One of the most important functions of boards of pharmacy is to protect the public health and welfare. Each state board must set standards of competence for the practice of pharmacy. State laws require the assessment of the proficiency of each candidate in the knowledge, skills, and abilities necessary for the practice of pharmacy. State boards use the NABPLEX to make that assessment. A candidate for licensure who passes this examination to the satisfaction of the relevant state board is judged to have the required proficiency in that state and can also practice pharmacy in other licensing jurisdictions.

The licensing examination, which is oriented toward professional practice, is a qualifying evaluation rather than a competitive test. The NABPLEX Review Committee has established standards of knowledge, skills, and abilities it considers essential for the practice of pharmacy. NABPLEX is used to assess these standards and is one determinant of a candidate's qualification for licensure. By its nature, the examination indicates that facts and information are meaningless without the ability to apply them in a practical situation. Furthermore, it highlights skills and abilities that must be maintained throughout the candidate's professional career.

Reciprocity Between States

Each state recognizes other states' licenses with the exceptions of California, Florida, and Hawaii, which require pharmacists to take their board of pharmacy examination before becoming licensed. The only requirement is that upon completing the state board of pharmacy requirements of a particular state, an individual must practice one year before being able to reciprocate his or her license from one state to another. Since Louisiana does not use the NABPLEX examination, some states may not honor the license from Louisiana and therefore require the student to take their board examination.

In order to reciprocate to another state, individuals must fill out the appropriate forms, which can be obtained from the National Association of Boards of Pharmacy and from the individual state board offices. Most state boards of pharmacy also require a law examination as well as the reciprocation papers. (The examination is on the federal and state laws governing pharmacy practice.) Specific information on reciprocation among various states can be obtained from the National Association of Boards of Pharmacy, One East Wacker Drive, Suite 2210, Chicago, Illinois, 60601, and/or the individual state board of pharmacy.

State Boards of Pharmacy

Alabama State Board of Pharmacy
1 Perimeter Park South, Suite 425 SO.
Birmingham, AL 35243
(205) 967-0130

Alaska State Board of Pharmacy
P.O. Box D—Lic
Juneau, AK 99811
(907) 465-2541

Arizona State Board of Pharmacy
5060 N. 19th Avenue, Suite 101
Phoenix, AZ 85015
(602) 255-5125

Arkansas State Board of Pharmacy
320 West Capital, Suite 802
Little Rock, AR 72201
(501) 371-3050

California State Board of Pharmacy
1020 N Street, Room 448
Sacramento, CA 95814
(916) 445-5014

Colorado State Board of Pharmacy
128 State Service Building
1525 Sherman
Denver, CO 80203

Connecticut Commission of Pharmacy
State Office Building, Room G-1A
Hartford, CT 06106
(203) 566-3917

Delaware State Board of Pharmacy
Robbins Building
802 Silver Lake Plaza
Dover, DE 19901
(302) 736-4708

District of Columbia Board of
  Pharmacy
614 H Street N.W. Room 923
Washington, DC 20001
(202) 727-7468

Florida Board of Pharmacy
130 North Monroe Street, Room 170
Tallahassee, FL 32399
(904) 488-7546

Georgia State Board of Pharmacy
State Examining Boards
166 Prior Street S.W.
Atlanta, GA 30303
(404) 656-9312

Hawaii State Board of Pharmacy
P.O. Box 3469
Honolulu, HI 96801
(808) 548-3086

Idaho Board of Pharmacy
500 South 10th Street
Boise, ID 83720
(208) 334-2356

Illinois Department of Professional
  Regulation
320 West Washington, 3rd Floor
Springfield, IL 62786
(217) 785-0800

Indiana Board of Pharmacy
Health Professions Bureau
One American Square, Suite 1020
P.O. Box 82067
Indianapolis, IN 46282
(317) 232-2960

Iowa Board of Pharmacy Examiners
1209 East Court, Executive Hills West
Des Moines, IA 50319
(515) 281-5944

Kansas State Board of Pharmacy
Landon State Office Building
900 Jackson, Room 513
Topeka, KS 66612
(913) 296-4056

Kentucky Board of Pharmacy
1228 U.S. 127 South
Frankfort, KY 40601
(502) 564-3833

Louisiana Board of Pharmacy
5615 Corporate Boulevard. Suite 8E
Baton Rouge, LA 70808
(504) 925-6496

Maine Board of Commissioners of
  Pharmacy
Department of Professional and
  Financial Regulation
Division of Licensing and Enforcement
Commission of Pharmacy, State House
  Station #35
Augusta, ME 04333
(207) 582-8723

Maryland Board of Pharmacy
4201 Patterson Avenue
Baltimore, MD 21215
(301) 764-4755

Massachusetts Board of Registration in
  Pharmacy
100 Cambridge Street, Room 1514
Boston, MA 02202
(617) 727-7390

Michigan Board of Pharmacy
611 West Ottawa, 4th Floor
P.O. Box 30018
Lansing, MI 48909
(517) 373-6873

Minnesota Board of Pharmacy
2700 University Avenue W, #107
St. Paul, MN 55114
(612) 642-0541

Mississippi State Board of Pharmacy
C&F Plaza, Suite 1165
2310 Highway 80 West
Jackson, MS 39204
(601) 354-6750

Missouri Board of Pharmacy
P.O. Box 625
Jefferson City, MO 65102
(314) 751-2334

Montana Board of Pharmacy
510 1st Avenue N., Suite 100
Great Falls, MT 59401
(406) 761-5131

Nebraska Board of Examiners in
  Pharmacy
P.O. Box 95007
Lincoln, NE 68509
(402) 471-2115

Nevada State Board of Pharmacy
1201 Terminal Way, Suite 212
Reno, NV 89502
(702) 322-0691

New Hampshire Board of Pharmacy
Health & Human Services Building
Hazen Drive
Concord, NH 03301
(603) 271-2350

New Jersey State Board of Pharmacy
1100 Raymond Boulevard
Newark, NJ 07102
(201) 648-2433

New Mexico Board of Pharmacy
4125 Carlisle N.E.
Albuquerque, NM 87107
(505) 841-6524

New York Board of Pharmacy
Cultural Education Center
Room 3035
Albany, NY 12230
(518) 474-3848

North Carolina Board of Pharmacy
P.O. Box 459
Carrboro, NC 27510
(919) 942-4454

North Dakota State Board of Pharmacy
P.O. Box 1354
Bismarck, ND 58502-1354
(701) 258-1535

Ohio State Board of Pharmacy
77 S. High Street, 17th floor
Columbus, OH 43266
(614) 466-4143

Oklahoma State Board of Pharmacy
4545 N. Lincoln Boulevard, Room 112
Oklahoma City, OK 73105
(405) 521-3815

Oregon State Board of Pharmacy
State Office Building, Room 505
1400 S.W. 5th
Portland, OR 97201
(503) 229-5849

Pennsylvania State Board of Pharmacy
Transportation & Safety Building, 6th
    Floor
P.O. 2649
Harrisburg, PA 17105
(717) 783-7157

Puerto Rico State Board of Pharmacy
Division of Exam Boards
Health Department—Pharmacy
Call Box 10,200
Santurce, PR 00908

Rhode Island Board of Pharmacy
Division of Drug Control
304 Cannon Building
75 Davis Street
Providence, RI 02908
(401) 277-2837

South Carolina Board of Pharmacy
P.O. Box 11927
Columbia, SC 29211
(803) 734-1010

South Dakota State Board of Pharmacy
P.O. Box 518
Pierre, SD 57501
(605) 244-2338

Tennessee Board of Pharmacy
Second Floor—Volunteer Plaza
500 James Robertson Parkway
Nashville, TN 37219
(615) 741-2718

Texas State Board of Pharmacy
8505 Cross Park Drive, Suite 110
Austin, TX 78754
(512) 832-0661

Utah Board of Pharmacy
160 East 300 South
P.O. Box 45802
Salt Lake City, UT 84145
(801) 530-6628

Vermont Board of Pharmacy
Pavilion Office Building
Montpelier, VT 05602
(802) 828-2372

Virginia Board of Pharmacy
1601 Rolling Hills Drive
Richmond, VA 23229
(804) 662-9911

Virgin Islands Board of Pharmacy
St. Thomas Hospital
48 Sugar Estate
St. Thomas, VI 00801
(809) 774-0117

Washington State Board of Pharmacy
WEA Building
319 East 7th Avenue—FF21
Olympia, WA 98504
(206) 753-6834

West Virginia Board of Pharmacy
150 Rockdale Road
Follansbee, WV 26037
(304) 527-1270

Wisconsin Pharmacy Examining
  Board
1400 East Washington
P.O. Box 8935
Madison, WI 53708
(608) 266-2811

Wyoming State Board of
  Pharmacy
1720 S. Poplar Street,
  Suite 5
Casper, WY 82601
(307) 234-0294

Requirements for Relicensure

Requirements for relicensure in some states only involve filling out the appropriate forms from the board of pharmacy and sending a check for your licensure fee each year. However, over the past several years, many states have started to require mandatory continuing education. As of October, 1989, 43 of the 50 states require continuing education for relicensure. These states are the following:

Alabama	Kentucky	New Mexico
Alaska	Louisiana	North Carolina
Arizona	Maine	North Dakota
Arkansas	Maryland	Ohio
California	Massachusetts	Oklahoma
Connecticut	Michigan	Oregon
Delaware	Minnesota	Pennsylvania
District of Columbia	Mississippi	Puerto Rico
Florida	Missouri	Rhode Island
Georgia	Montana	South Carolina
Idaho	Nebraska	South Dakota
Illinois	Nevada	Tennessee
Indiana	New Hampshire	Washington
Iowa	New Jersey	Wyoming
Kansas		

The numbers of hours of continuing education that are required range from a minimum of ten hours (contact hours) per year up to thirty contact hours every two years. Continuing education credits are defined in the following manner: one continuing education unit (1.0 CEU) equals ten contact hours of credit. Pharmacists are required to report the continuing education programs attended to their board of pharmacy.

The ACPE approves providers of pharmacy continuing education. The provider approval program assures pharmacists of the quality of continuing education programs by evaluating the capability of the providers of activities. Its aims are the following:

1. Advance the quality of continuing education, thereby assisting in the advancement of the practice of pharmacy.

2. Establish criteria and characteristics of approved continuing pharmaceutical education programs.

3. Provide pharmacists with a dependable basis for selecting continuing education programs.

4. Provide a basis for uniform acceptance of continuing education credits among the states.

5. Provide feedback of information to providers about their offerings, encouraging periodic self-evaluation with a view toward continual improvement and strengthening of continuing education activities.

A pamphlet describing the standards for assessing and approving continuing education programs, as well as a list of approved continuing education programs, can be obtained from the American Council on Pharmaceutical Education, One East Wacker Drive, Suite 2210, Chicago, Illinois 60601.

PART FOUR

PCAT REVIEW

Introduction to the PCAT

About the Test

The Pharmacy College Admission Test (PCAT) is designed to measure the general ability and scientific knowledge of applicants seeking admission to selected pharmacy programs. The PCAT is developed and administered by the Psychological Corporation, under the auspices of the American Association of Colleges of Pharmacy. The test is generally given three times a year; scores are available about four weeks after the test date. It currently costs $30.00 to take the PCAT, receive your scores, and have your scores forwarded to up to three different colleges of pharmacy if you are a preregistered applicant for the exam.

Further information concerning registration for the PCAT may be obtained by writing to:

Pharmacy College Admission Test
The Psychological Corporation
555 Academic Court
San Antonio, TX 78204

or by calling The Psychological Corporation at (512) 554-8198.

Examination Contents

The PCAT is divided into five areas:

Verbal Ability—General, nonscientific word knowledge, typically indicative of academic aptitude.

Quantitative Ability—A combination of assessment of skills in arithmetic processes including fractions, decimals, and percentages, and of ability to reason through and understand quantitative concepts and relationships, including applications of algebra but not of trigonometry or calculus.

Biology—Survey of principles and concepts in basic biology with major emphasis on human biology.

Chemistry—Sampling of problems and principles in inorganic and elementary organic chemistry.

Reading Comprehension—Ability to comprehend, analyze, understand, and interpret the contents of reading passages on scientific topics.

There is a total of about four hours of testing time. The test consists of objective, multiple-choice questions, and there is only one right answer for each. No examinee is expected to answer all the questions correctly. Scores are based on the number of right answers only; there is no penalty for guessing.

Answer Sheet
Verbal Ability

1 ① ② ③ ④   21 ① ② ③ ④   41 ① ② ③ ④   61 ① ② ③ ④   81 ① ② ③ ④

2 ① ② ③ ④   22 ① ② ③ ④   42 ① ② ③ ④   62 ① ② ③ ④   82 ① ② ③ ④

3 ① ② ③ ④   23 ① ② ③ ④   43 ① ② ③ ④   63 ① ② ③ ④   83 ① ② ③ ④

4 ① ② ③ ④   24 ① ② ③ ④   44 ① ② ③ ④   64 ① ② ③ ④   84 ① ② ③ ④

5 ① ② ③ ④   25 ① ② ③ ④   45 ① ② ③ ④   65 ① ② ③ ④   85 ① ② ③ ④

6 ① ② ③ ④   26 ① ② ③ ④   46 ① ② ③ ④   66 ① ② ③ ④   86 ① ② ③ ④

7 ① ② ③ ④   27 ① ② ③ ④   47 ① ② ③ ④   67 ① ② ③ ④   87 ① ② ③ ④

8 ① ② ③ ④   28 ① ② ③ ④   48 ① ② ③ ④   68 ① ② ③ ④   88 ① ② ③ ④

9 ① ② ③ ④   29 ① ② ③ ④   49 ① ② ③ ④   69 ① ② ③ ④   89 ① ② ③ ④

10 ① ② ③ ④   30 ① ② ③ ④   50 ① ② ③ ④   70 ① ② ③ ④   90 ① ② ③ ④

11 ① ② ③ ④   31 ① ② ③ ④   51 ① ② ③ ④   71 ① ② ③ ④   91 ① ② ③ ④

12 ① ② ③ ④   32 ① ② ③ ④   52 ① ② ③ ④   72 ① ② ③ ④   92 ① ② ③ ④

13 ① ② ③ ④   33 ① ② ③ ④   53 ① ② ③ ④   73 ① ② ③ ④   93 ① ② ③ ④

14 ① ② ③ ④   34 ① ② ③ ④   54 ① ② ③ ④   74 ① ② ③ ④   94 ① ② ③ ④

15 ① ② ③ ④   35 ① ② ③ ④   55 ① ② ③ ④   75 ① ② ③ ④   95 ① ② ③ ④

16 ① ② ③ ④   36 ① ② ③ ④   56 ① ② ③ ④   76 ① ② ③ ④   96 ① ② ③ ④

17 ① ② ③ ④   37 ① ② ③ ④   57 ① ② ③ ④   77 ① ② ③ ④   97 ① ② ③ ④

18 ① ② ③ ④   38 ① ② ③ ④   58 ① ② ③ ④   78 ① ② ③ ④   98 ① ② ③ ④

19 ① ② ③ ④   39 ① ② ③ ④   59 ① ② ③ ④   79 ① ② ③ ④   99 ① ② ③ ④

20 ① ② ③ ④   40 ① ② ③ ④   60 ① ② ③ ④   80 ① ② ③ ④   100 ① ② ③ ④

VERBAL ABILITY

100 Questions   1 Hour, 40 Minutes

Directions: Choose the numbered word that means the <u>same</u> or most nearly the same as the word in capital letters.

1. EXTENT *étendue*

    1. exterior
    2. width *largeurs*
    3. limit
    4. justification

2. AWAKE

    1. arouse
    2. sleep
    3. drowse
    4. supply

3. TACT

    1. act
    2. diplomacy
    3. enactment
    4. expert

4. EXPERT

    1. amateur
    2. feat
    3. authority
    4. neophyte

5. ACCOUNT

    1. bookkeeper
    2. count
    3. basis
    4. statement

6. ACCRUE

    1. acquire
    2. accumulate
    3. chaw
    4. achieve

7. BULLETIN

    1. announcement
    2. board
    3. newt
    4. bullet

8. BRIDLE

    1. bridge
    2. bride
    3. control
    4. center

9. CONTAMINATE

    1. pollute
    2. contemplate
    3. contain
    4. purify

10. DISPLEASURE

    1. pique
    2. disposal
    3. madness
    4. bitterness

11. EVENTUATE

1. end
2. entwine
3. crease
4. ensue

12. MAGNIFICENCE

1. fame
2. magnifier
3. grandiosity
4. magnitude

13. UNDULATE

1. poll
2. slither
3. retreat
4. retch

14. PARSIMONIOUS

1. niggardly
2. liberal
3. conservative
4. truest

15. QUIESCENT

1. mobile
2. running
3. immobile
4. motor

16. RADIOACTIVITY

1. radio
2. radiation
3. radar
4. ion

17. COLLEGIAN

1. group
2. colleague
3. student
4. classmate

18. FLANK

1. side
2. end
3. head
4. sirloin

19. DIPSOMANIAC *alcoholic*

1. sobriety
2. insomniac
3. alcoholic
4. addict

20. CORSAGE

1. butler
2. nosegay
3. receptionist
4. corset

21. CORTEGE

1. roadway
2. retinue
3. line
4. lineation

22. JOWL

1. head
2. pig
3. owl
4. jaw

23. SUPREMACY

1. headiness
2. chieftaincy
3. secondary
4. super

24. PLIABLE

1. flexible
2. scrupulous
3. programmable
4. reliable

25. ZEALOT

1. nut
2. fanatic
3. crazy
4. zany

26. TRANSCEND

1. overtake
2. pass
3. exceed
4. send

27. SHREWD

    1. cagey
    2. odd
    3. shrinkable
    4. crooked

28. EXPENDITURE

    1. credit
    2. disbursement
    3. debit
    4. ovolo

29. EXPEDIENCY

    1. expellee
    2. expulsion
    3. efficiency
    4. appropriateness

30. SILKEN

    1. worm-eaten
    2. woolen
    3. luxurious
    4. sulky

31. DEPART

    1. withdraw
    2. relieve
    3. repass
    4. report

32. DENOUNCE

    1. eulogize
    2. impeach
    3. connote
    4. express

33. DENUDE

    1. peel
    2. deodorize
    3. depart
    4. deperm

34. FLYSPECK

    1. mot
    2. circle
    3. speckle
    4. hang

35. DEVIATORY

    1. aberrant
    2. normal
    3. nontitled
    4. ghostly

36. MELEE

    1. agreement
    2. melange
    3. skirmish
    4. melilot

37. MEDICAMENT

    1. medium
    2. medicine
    3. herb
    4. law

38. PALPABLE

    1. pulpy
    2. palmary
    3. touchable
    4. tactful

39. RUDIMENTARY

    1. parcel
    2. mathematical
    3. parietal
    4. basal

40. TONICITY

    1. tone
    2. tonus
    3. tonic
    4. care

41. VALIDATE

    1. abrogate
    2. cancel
    3. authenticate
    4. abolish

42. TARIFF

    1. post
    2. senior
    3. goal
    4. duty

43. WARBLE

   1. tone
   2. diapason
   3. sin
   4. waddle

44. YAHOO

   1. yak
   2. ruffian
   3. blabber
   4. chat

45. SUAVE

   1. bluff
   2. foolish
   3. urbane
   4. urban

46. REMORSELESS

   1. impenitent
   2. remorseful
   3. remorsefully
   4. regretful

47. PERSNICKETY

   1. easy
   2. pernicious
   3. chancy
   4. fastidious

48. PERIMETER

   1. period
   2. periphery
   3. area
   4. end zone

49. IMPERIOUS

   1. kindly
   2. gentle
   3. considerate
   4. domineering

50. COMPASSION

   1. unconcern
   2. implacability
   3. relentlessness
   4. clemency

Directions: Choose the numbered word that means the opposite or most nearly the opposite to the word in capital letters.

51. DIFFICULTY

   1. hardship
   2. burden
   3. trouble
   4. effortlessness

52. IDEALISM

   1. utopianism
   2. realism
   3. romanticism
   4. perfectionism

53. HYSTERICAL

   1. overwrought
   2. calm
   3. worked up
   4. crazy

54. WELCOME

   1. hello
   2. goodbye
   3. greeting
   4. salutation

55. SILVER

   1. gold
   2. nickel
   3. iron
   4. xenon

56. EXTRANEOUS

   1. alien
   2. foreign
   3. extrinsic
   4. intrinsic

57. FACTORY

   1. plant
   2. workshop
   3. store
   4. manufacturer

58. TAME

   1. docile
   2. submissive
   3. calm
   4. fierce

59. MAELSTROM

   1. whirl
   2. steadiness
   3. fury
   4. storm

60. NEFARIOUS

   1. corrupt
   2. degenerate
   3. generous
   4. putrid

61. OPINION

   1. view
   2. operation
   3. belief
   4. persuasion

62. PARALLEL

   1. vertical
   2. analogous
   3. correlative
   4. equivalent

63. QUASH

   1. abrogate
   2. dissolve
   3. initiate
   4. quell

64. QUAY

   1. jetty
   2. levee
   3. pier
   4. harbor

65 ANIMATION

   1. rebirth
   2. evisceration
   3. risorgimento
   4. revivification

66. REMONSTRATION

   1. challenge
   2. acquiescence
   3. difficulty
   4. demurral

67. ECLECTIC

   1. selective
   2. discriminating
   3. picky
   4. homogeneous

68. FAMOUS

   1. undistinguished
   2. celebrated
   3. redoubtable
   4. prestigious

69. GLUTTONOUS

   1. edacious
   2. rapacious
   3. abstemious
   4. ravenous

70. GLOAMING

   1. evening
   2. morning
   3. twilight
   4. eventide

71. GNOME

   1. aphorism
   2. human
   3. apothegm
   4. brocard

72. GLIMPSE

   1. gander
   2. glance
   3. peek
   4. peer

73. GLOOMY

    1. gloomless
    2. mirthless
    3. lightless
    4. murky

74. INTONATION

    1. tone
    2. accent
    3. inflection
    4. inarticulateness

75. JOVIALITY

    1. mirth
    2. hilarity
    3. melancholy
    4. jollity

76. SAGE

    1. savant
    2. temerariousness
    3. scholar
    4. wiseman

77. LISSOME

    1. rigid
    2. supple
    3. lithe
    4. limber

78. OBDURATE

    1. callous
    2. coldhearted
    3. tender
    4. mulish

79. OBSTREPEROUS

    1. blatant
    2. whist
    3. clamorous
    4. vociferous

80. VALEDICTION

    1. epistle
    2. generosity
    3. greeting
    4. insecurity

81. OPEN-AIR

    1. outside
    2. inside
    3. alfresco
    4. outdoor

82. HUMANOID

    1. anthropoid
    2. anthropomorphic
    3. anthropological
    4. animal-like

83. BUOYANCY

    1. ebullience
    2. effervescence
    3. sinkage
    4. exuberancy

84. BURG

    1. camp
    2. village
    3. city
    4. municipality

85. ENTHRALLED

    1. flimsy
    2. empty
    3. free
    4. weak

86. SENILE

    1. keen
    2. ancient
    3. senescent
    4. decrepit

87. TELESTHETIC

    1. mystical
    2. telephonic
    3. mystic
    4. anagogic

88. TEMERITY

    1. daredevil
    2. caution
    3. venturer
    4. audacity

89. POLYCHROMATIC

1. variegated
2. parti-colored
3. versicolored
4. monochromatic

90. MODIFY

1. change
2. alter
3. vary
4. continue

91. FURORE

1. ado
2. applause
3. stir
4. whirl

92. CONCILIATE

1. antagonize
2. pacify
3. appease
4. reconcile

93. DESCENDANT

1. kin
2. ancestor
3. seed
4. progeny

94. FAIR

1. just
2. equitable
3. unbiased
4. biased

95. LASCIVIOUS

1. lewd
2. libertine
3. puritan
4. salacious

96. PURCHASABLE

1. marketable
2. salable
3. unavailable
4. obtainable

97. RESTITUTE

1. reclaim
2. take
3. rejuvenate
4. recover

98. MEDLEY

1. hodgepodge
2. uniform
3. jumbled
4. mixed

99. IMPROMPTU

1. planless
2. extemporaneous
3. improvisational
4. rehearsed

100. WHIMSICAL

1. vagarious
2. whimsied
3. steadfast
4. capricious

Answer Sheet
Quantitative Ability

101 ① ② ③ ④   121 ① ② ③ ④   141 ① ② ③ ④   161 ① ② ③ ④   181 ① ② ③ ④

102 ① ② ③ ④   122 ① ② ③ ④   142 ① ② ③ ④   162 ① ② ③ ④   182 ① ② ③ ④

103 ① ② ③ ④   123 ① ② ③ ④   143 ① ② ③ ④   163 ① ② ③ ④   183 ① ② ③ ④

104 ① ② ③ ④   124 ① ② ③ ④   144 ① ② ③ ④   164 ① ② ③ ④   184 ① ② ③ ④

105 ① ② ③ ④   125 ① ② ③ ④   145 ① ② ③ ④   165 ① ② ③ ④   185 ① ② ③ ④

106 ① ② ③ ④   126 ① ② ③ ④   146 ① ② ③ ④   166 ① ② ③ ④   186 ① ② ③ ④

107 ① ② ③ ④   127 ① ② ③ ④   147 ① ② ③ ④   167 ① ② ③ ④   187 ① ② ③ ④

108 ① ② ③ ④   128 ① ② ③ ④   148 ① ② ③ ④   168 ① ② ③ ④   188 ① ② ③ ④

109 ① ② ③ ④   129 ① ② ③ ④   149 ① ② ③ ④   169 ① ② ③ ④   189 ① ② ③ ④

110 ① ② ③ ④   130 ① ② ③ ④   150 ① ② ③ ④   170 ① ② ③ ④   190 ① ② ③ ④

111 ① ② ③ ④   131 ① ② ③ ④   151 ① ② ③ ④   171 ① ② ③ ④   191 ① ② ③ ④

112 ① ② ③ ④   132 ① ② ③ ④   152 ① ② ③ ④   172 ① ② ③ ④   192 ① ② ③ ④

113 ① ② ③ ④   133 ① ② ③ ④   153 ① ② ③ ④   173 ① ② ③ ④   193 ① ② ③ ④

114 ① ② ③ ④   134 ① ② ③ ④   154 ① ② ③ ④   174 ① ② ③ ④   194 ① ② ③ ④

115 ① ② ③ ④   135 ① ② ③ ④   155 ① ② ③ ④   175 ① ② ③ ④   195 ① ② ③ ④

116 ① ② ③ ④   136 ① ② ③ ④   156 ① ② ③ ④   176 ① ② ③ ④   196 ① ② ③ ④

117 ① ② ③ ④   137 ① ② ③ ④   157 ① ② ③ ④   177 ① ② ③ ④   197 ① ② ③ ④

118 ① ② ③ ④   138 ① ② ③ ④   158 ① ② ③ ④   178 ① ② ③ ④   198 ① ② ③ ④

119 ① ② ③ ④   139 ① ② ③ ④   159 ① ② ③ ④   179 ① ② ③ ④   199 ① ② ③ ④

120 ① ② ③ ④   140 ① ② ③ ④   160 ① ② ③ ④   180 ① ② ③ ④   200 ① ② ③ ④

QUANTITATIVE ABILITY

100 Questions   2 Hours

Directions: Choose the best answer to each of the following questions.

101. $\frac{3}{8} + \frac{4}{5} =$

    1. $\frac{95}{80}$

    2. 1.2

    3. $1\frac{7}{40}$

    4. $\frac{12}{40}$

102. $0.25 + \frac{15}{16} =$

    1. 1.08

    2. $1\frac{3}{16}$

    3. 3.75

    4. $\frac{24}{16}$

103. $1.30 \times 236 =$

    1. 3.068×10^2

    2. 3068×10^1

    3. 283.2

    4. 29.9×10^2

104. log(50 x 2) =

    1. (log 50) x (log 2)

    2. (log 2) x (10 log 5)

    3. log 10

    4. log 2 + log 50

105. log 0.001 =

    1. 3

    2. 100

    3. -3

    4. $\frac{1}{3}$

106. $\sqrt[3]{8}$ =

    1. 2^3

    2. $\frac{8}{2}$

    3. $8^{\frac{1}{3}}$

    4. 8 log 3

107. $\log_{10} 1000$ =

    1. 10

    2. 3

3. 100

4. 4

108. $1 \times 10^{-2} + 2.3 \times 10^1$

   1. 2.3×10^2

   2. 24.0

   3. 23.01

   4. 23.1

109. $\frac{3}{16} =$

   1. 25%

   2. $\frac{9}{32}$

   3. 18.75%

   4. 33%

110. $\frac{(2.3\ g)}{(10\ ml)} =$

   1. 2.3%

   2. 0.23%

   3. 23% wt/vol

   4. 2.3/100

111. How many liters of a 4% solution can be made from 24 g of a drug?

    1. 6 liters

    2. 0.6 liter

    3. 0.096 liter

    4. 96 liters

112. How much 0.9% NaCl can be made from 1 liter of an 18% stock solution of NaCl?

    1. 0.05 liter

    2. 5.0 liters

    3. 2.0 liters

    4. 20 liters

113. What is the percentage of ethanol in a mixture composed of 5 liters of 25%, 2 liters of 50%, and 0.5 liter of 10% ethanol?

    1. 11.3%

    2. 50%

    3. 30.7%

    4. 22%

114. $\log \sqrt{25}$

    1. $\frac{1}{2} \log 25$

    2. $\log 25^{\frac{1}{2}}$

3. log 5

4. all of the above

115. log 25^2

1. log 50

2. 5

3. log 5

4. 2 log 25

116. If 1 kg equals 2.2 lb, how many grams are in 1 lb?

1. 454.5 g

2. 2200 g

3. 97.8 g

4. 1200 g

117. Subtract 283 ml from 1 liter.

1. 217 ml

2. 9717 ml

3. 717 ml

4. none of the above

118. If 15.43 grains are in 1 g, how many milligrams equals 1 grain?

    1. 0.065 mg

    2. 984.6 mg

    3. 84.57 mg

    4. 64.81 mg

119. $\sqrt[3]{3^6} + \sqrt{2^2} =$

    1. 7

    2. 11

    3. 36

    4. none of the above

120. $\left(\dfrac{2}{3}\right)^2 + 2^{-3} =$

    1. $\dfrac{41}{72}$

    2. $\dfrac{4}{48}$

    3. $\dfrac{2}{24}$

    4. $\dfrac{2}{3}$

121. $10° + 10^1 + 10^{-1} =$

    1. 10.1

    2. 101

3.   11.1

4.   1.1

122.   If 9(X°C) = 5(Y°F) - 160, what is 79°F in degrees centigrade?

1.   23.5°C

2.   87.1°C

3.   26.1°C

4.   174.2°C

123.   What is -10°C in degrees Fahrenheit?

1.   50°F

2.   14°F

3.   -12.2°F

4.   -10°F

124.   If the temperature dropped from 72 to 65°F, how many degrees centigrade change was there?

1.   7°C

2.   13.9°C

3.   44.6°C

4.   3.9°C

125. How much substance is needed for 200 ml of a 1:10,000 solution?

    1. 1 g

    2. 200 mg

    3. 0.02 g

    4. 2 mg

Refer to the following graph for Questions 126-130.

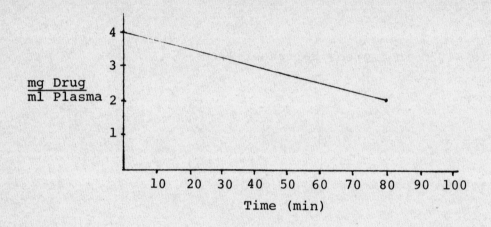

126. At 20 min, how much drug remained in the plasma?

    1. 2 mg/ml

    2. There was no change.

    3. 3.5 mg/ml

    4. cannot be determined from graph

127. At what rate is the drug disappearing from the plasma?

    1. 2 mg/ml plasma per 60 min

    2. 4 mg/ml plasma per 80 min

    3. 1.5 mg/ml plasma per hour

    4. none of the above

128. At 2 hr what would be the concentration of drug in the plasma?

    1. 0.5 mg/ml

    2. 1 mg/ml

    3. No drug will remain.

    4. none of the above

129. If the initial drug concentration had been 8 mg/ml and the rate of disappearance stayed the same, what would have been the drug concentration at 80 min?

    1. 6 mg/ml

    2. 4 mg/ml

    3. 2 mg/ml

    4. none of the above

130. How long would it take the drug concentration to reach 0 mg/ml if the initial concentration was 4 mg/ml?

    1. 2 hr

    2. 200 min

3. 160 min

4. 150 min

For Questions 131 and 132, find all positive <u>integers</u> satisfying the inequality.

131. $4 < 3\underline{x} - 2 \leq 10$

    1. 5, 6, 7, 8, 9, 10

    2. 1, 2, 3

    3. 3, 4

    4. none of the above

132. $\dfrac{7}{\underline{x}} > 2$, with $\underline{x} \neq 0$

    1. 7

    2. 1, 2, 3

    3. 2, 7

    4. none of the above

133. $|-5| - |-2| =$

    1. -3

    2. 7

    3. 3

    4. -7

134. $|8| - |14|$

   1. 6

   2. -6

   3. 22

   4. none of the above

135. Solve $|5\underline{x} + 4| = -3$ for $\underline{x}$.

   1. $\dfrac{7}{5}$

   2. $\dfrac{1}{5}$

   3. 2

   4. none of the above

Refer to the following diagram for Questions 136-138.

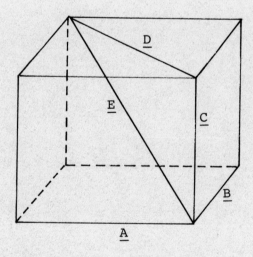

   $\underline{A} = \underline{B} = \underline{C}$ $\underline{A} = 2$ in.

136. What is the length of line <u>D</u>?

    1. 2 in.

    2. $\sqrt{8}$ in.

    3. 4 in.

    4. $\sqrt{5}$ in.

137. What is the area encompassed by lines <u>C</u>, <u>D</u>, and <u>E</u>?

    1. $\sqrt{8}$ in.^{2}

    2. $2\sqrt{3}$ in.^{2}

    3. 2 in.^{2}

    4. 4 in.^{2}

138. What is the total surface area of the cube?

    1. 24 in.^{2}

    2. 16 in.^{2}

    3. 12 in.^{2}

    4. 32 in.^{2}

Refer to the following diagram for Questions 139-142.

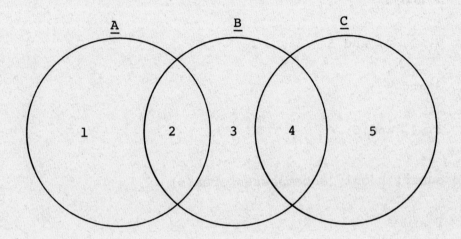

139. The subset "<u>A</u> or <u>B</u>" encompasses area(s)

1. 1 and 3

2. 2

3. 1, 2, and 3

4. 1, 2, 3, and 4

140. The subset "<u>A</u> and <u>B</u>" encompasses area(s)

1. 1 and 3

2. 2

3. 1, 2, and 3

4. 1, 2, 3, and 4

141. The subset "<u>A</u> or <u>C</u>, but not <u>B</u>" encompasses area(s)

1. 1 and 5

2. 1, 2, 4, and 5

3. 2 and 4

4. 1, 4, and 5

142. The subset <u>B</u> only encompasses area(s)

1. 1 and 3

2. 2, 3, and 4

3. 2 and 4

4. 3

Refer to the following diagrams for Questions 143-145.

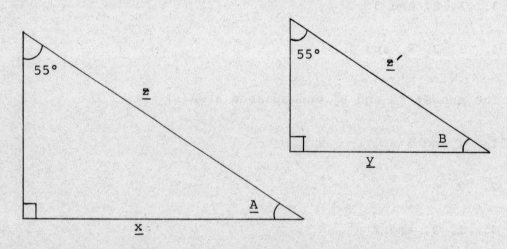

143. If x = 2y, what is the ratio of the areas of the two triangles (x:y)?

    1. 2:1

    2. 4:1

    3. 1:2

    4. $\sqrt{2}$:1

144. How many degrees are there in angle A?

    1. 60°

    2. 45°

    3. 90°

    4. 35°

145. If x = 3y and z = 5, what is z'?

    1. $\sqrt{5}$

    2. 3

    3. $\frac{3}{5}$

    4. $1\frac{2}{3}$

Refer to the following graph for Questions 146 and 147.

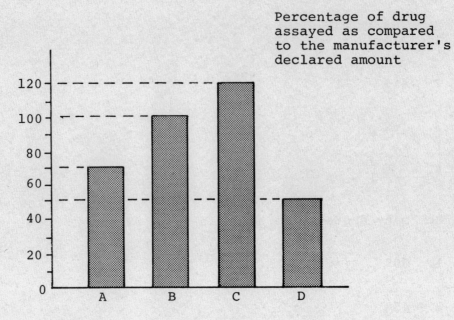

Percentage of drug assayed as compared to the manufacturer's declared amount

146. If a minimum of 90% of the declared amount of active drug is required by law, which drugs may be used?

    1. C only

    2. B and C

    3. A, B, and C

    4. none of the above

147. If the amount of drug declared by the manufacturer was 200 mg, how much drug was present in the drug samples accepted in the previous question?

    1. 200 mg

    2. 100 and 120 mg

3. 200 and 240 mg

4. none of the above

Refer to the following graph for Questions 148-150.

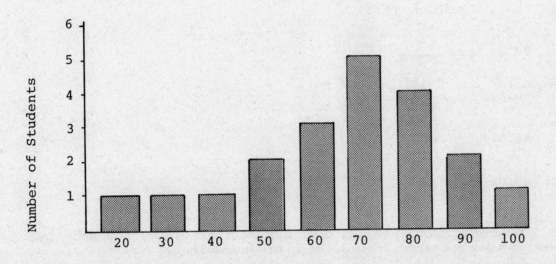

Scores on final exam
(percent)

148. What is the mean percent score for the final exam?

1. 70.0%

2. 60.0%

3. 66.0%

4. 80.0%

149. What is the modal score?

1. 70.0%

   2. 60.0%

   3. 66.0%

   4. 80.0%

150. What is the median score?

   1. 70.0%

   2. 60.0%

   3. 66.0%

   4. 80.0%

151. If 50 tablets contain 0.625 g of active ingredient, how many tablets can be prepared from 31.25 g of ingredient?

   1. 2500 tablets

   2. 25 tablets

   3. 625 tablets

   4. 100 tablets

152. The adult (weight, 150 lb) dose of a drug is 70 μg. Approximately what is the dose for a child weighing 44 lb?

   1. 200 μg

   2. 20 μg

   3. 3 μg

   4. none of the above

153. If $\underline{x} = 1/\underline{y}$, what happens to $\underline{y}$ when $\underline{x}$ is increased to $2\underline{x}$?

   1. $\underline{y}$ increases by a factor of 2

   2. $\underline{y}$ decreases by a factor of ½

   3. There is no change in $\underline{y}$

   4. $\underline{y}$ increases by a factor of 4

154. If $\underline{x} = 2\underline{y}$, what happens to $\underline{y}$ when $\underline{x}$ is increased to $2\underline{x}$?

   1. $\underline{y}$ increases by a factor of 2

   2. $\underline{y}$ decreases by a factor of ½

   3. There is no change in $\underline{y}$

   4. $\underline{y}$ increases by a factor of 4

155. A quantity of drug weighing 24 g is divided into 16 equal parts. How much does each part weigh?

   1. 150 mg

   2. 2666 mg

   3. 0.150 g

   4. 1500 mg

156. If there may be a 10% error in the weight of a tablet, what is the range of acceptable tablet weights when a tablet of 150 g is desired?

   1. 135-150 g

   2. 140-160 g

3. 130-170 g

4. 135-165 g

157. If there are 65 mg of elemental iron in 325 mg of ferrous sulfate, what percentage of the tablet weight is due to the iron?

1. 20%

2. 2%

3. 5%

4. 50%

158. A compound has a maximal solubility of 50 mg/ml. How much is needed to make a 1 liter solution at the maximal concentration?

1. 5000 mg

2. 20 g

3. 1000 mg

4. 50 g

159. If a graduated cylinder is marked in 5-ml intervals, what is the smallest volume that can be measured with a 10% error?

1. 5 ml

2. 50 ml

3. 100 ml

4. 10 ml

160. Give the average of the following to the nearest whole number: 61, 50, 100, 50.

    1. 50

    2. 65

    3. 55

    4. cannot be determined

Refer to the following graph for Questions 161-163.

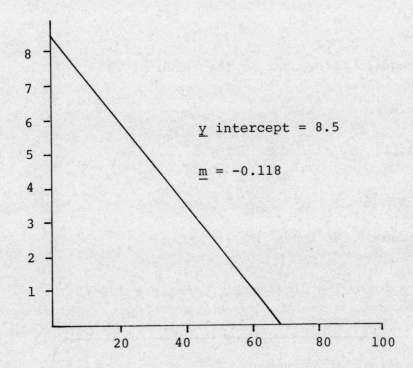

y intercept = 8.5

$\underline{m}$ = -0.118

161. What is the equation for the line?

    1. $\underline{y}$ = 8.5 + 0.118$\underline{x}$

    2. 8.5$\underline{y}$ = 0.118$\underline{x}$

3. $y = -0.118x + 8.5$

4. $y = -0.118x/8.5$

162. If y equals 6, what is the value of x to the nearest whole number?

   1. 21

   2. 40

   3. 123

   4. 10

163. If x equals zero, what is the value of y?

   1. 0.0

   2. 0.118

   3. 8.5

   4. none of the above

Refer to the following diagram for Questions 164-166.

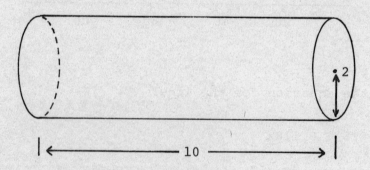

164. What is the volume of the cylinder ($\pi \cong 3.14$)?

    1. 987 cubic units

    2. 314 cubic units

    3. 126 cubic units

    4. 63 cubic units

165. What is the lateral surface area of the cylinder?

    1. 987 square units

    2. 314 square units

    3. 126 square units

    4. 63 square units

166. What is the total surface area?

    1. 314 square units

    2. 151 square units

    3. 126 square units

    4. 135 square units

167.

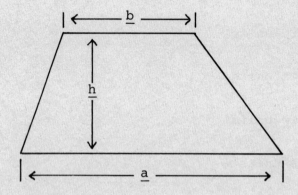

What is the area of the trapezoid when a = 4, b = 2, and h = 1?

1. 4 square units

2. 3 square units

3. 6 square units

4. 8 square units

168.

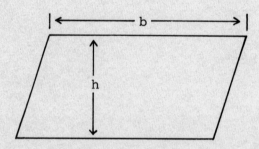

What is the area of the parallelogram when $\underline{b}$ = 5 and $\underline{h}$ = 2 ?

1. 5 square units

2. 20 square units

3. 10 square units

4. 2.5 square units

169. If $\underline{y}$ = 3$\underline{a}$ + $\underline{b}$ and $\underline{x}$ = 3$\underline{b}$ + $\underline{a}$, find $\underline{y}$ in terms of $\underline{x}$ and $\underline{b}$.

1. 3$\underline{b}$ + 8$\underline{x}$

2. 3$\underline{b}$ - 8$\underline{x}$

3. 3$\underline{x}$ - 8$\underline{b}$

4. 3$\underline{x}$ + 8$\underline{b}$

170. Given the equation $\underline{y}$ = $\underline{mx}$ + $\underline{c}$, a linear plot of $\underline{y}$ versus $\underline{x}$ will yield

1. a slope of $\underline{m}$

2. an ordinate intercept of 1/$\underline{c}$

3. an abscissa intercept of $\underline{c}$

4. all of the above

171. $\dfrac{7 \div 3}{21 \div 3}$ =

1. $\dfrac{7}{21}$

2. $\frac{1}{3}$

3. 0.33

4. all of the above

172. Reduce $\frac{72}{2880}$ to lowest terms

1. $\frac{1}{120}$

2. $\frac{1}{124}$

3. $\frac{1}{52}$

4. $\frac{1}{40}$

173. A prescription calls for 7.5 mg of a drug. How many tablets containing 0.25 mg of the drug are required?

1. 30

2. 31

3. 15

4. 17

174. Add $\frac{3}{4}$ mg, 0.25 mg, $\frac{2}{5}$ mg, and 2.75 mg.

1. 5.0 mg

2. 4.0 mg

3. 4.15 mg

4. 5.15 mg

175.   Add 0.75 mg, 50 g, and 0.5 kg.

       1.   550.00075 g

       2.   500.75 g

       3.   0.5575 kg

       4.   500,575 mg

176. $3\frac{1}{8}$ is the same as

       1. $\frac{75}{36}$

       2. $\frac{100}{32}$

       3. $\frac{125}{32}$

       4. $\frac{125}{36}$

177.   If 60 mg = 1 grain, then 10% of 360 mg =

       1.   6 grain

       2.   0.6 grain

       3.   0.06 grain

       4.   60 grain

178. $2\sqrt{36} + \dfrac{4\sqrt{28}}{3\sqrt{7}} =$

       1. $14\sqrt{7}$

2. $12\frac{2}{3}$

3. $13\sqrt{7}$

4. $14\frac{2}{3}$

179. If $\underline{A} = e^{\underline{a}}$, then $1 + \underline{A} =$

1. $1 + e^{\underline{a}}$

2. $e^{\underline{a}}$

3. $1/e^{\underline{a}}$

4. $\ln e^{\underline{a}}$

180. $7.7 \times 10° =$

1. 0

2. 0.77

3. 7.7

4. 77

181. $1,000,000$ can also be expressed as

1. $1 \times 10^6 \times 10^1$

2. $1 \times 10^3 \times 10^{-3}$

3. $1 \times 10^3 \times 10^3$

4. $1 \times 10^6 \times 10^{-3}$

182. $\sqrt{144 \times 10^4} =$

    1. 2400

    2. 800

    3. 1600

    4. 1200

183. If 1 kg = 2.2 lb, add the following and express the answer in kilograms: 132 lb, 11 lb, and 44 lb.

    1. 85 kg

    2. 88 kg

    3. 98 kg

    4. 58 kg

184. $\left(\dfrac{3}{4}\right)^2 + 3^2 + \sqrt{\dfrac{49}{256}} =$

    1. 27

    2. 10.0

    3. 29

    4. 30

185. A given line has a slope of -2 and a y intercept (0, $\sqrt{2}$). It can be expressed as the linear equation

    1. $y = -2x$

    2. $y = \sqrt{2} + 2x$

3. $\underline{y} = -2\underline{x} + \sqrt{2}$

4. $\underline{y} = 2\underline{x}$

186. Find the value of $\dfrac{250,000 \times 0.018}{0.15}$

1. 300,000

2. 275,000

3. 37,000

4. 30,000

187. What is $\underline{x}$ if $\underline{x}^{-3} = \dfrac{1}{27}$?

1. 3

2. $\dfrac{1}{3}$

3. 0.6

4. 9

188. What is $\underline{I}$?

1. $\underline{KH}/\underline{J}$

2. $\underline{JH}/\underline{K}$

3. $\underline{JK}/\underline{H}$

4. none of the above

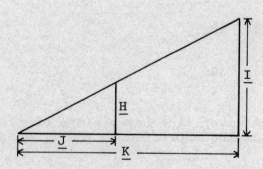

Questions 189-193 refer to the following statement:

A compound is composed (by weight) of drug A, 20%; drug B, 5%; and drug C, 75%.

189. What amount of drug A is required to make 500 g of the compound?

1. 100 g

2. 125 g

3. 375 g

4. 400 g

190. What amount of the drugs A and B is needed to make 500 g of the compound?

1. 100 g

2. 125 g

3. 375 g

4. 400 g

191. What amount of the drugs B and C is needed to make 500 g of the compound?

1. 100 g

2. 125 g

3. 375 g

4. 400 g

192. What amount of the drugs A, B, and C is needed to make 100 g of the compound?

    1. 100 g

    2. 125 g

    3. 375 g

    4. 400 g

193. What are the ratios A:B:C as indicated in the formula?

    1. 4:15:1

    2. 4:1:15

    3. 15:1:4

    4. none of the above

194. Given that $\dfrac{(B - p)}{q} = \dfrac{(g_a/M_a)}{g_b/M_b}$, find g_b.

    1. $\dfrac{B - p}{q} \quad \dfrac{M_a M_b}{g_a}$

    2. $\dfrac{p - B}{q} \quad \dfrac{M_b g_a}{M_a}$

    3. $\dfrac{q}{B - p} \quad M_b M_a g_a$

    4. $\dfrac{q}{B - p} \quad \dfrac{M_b g_a}{M_a}$

195. Consider the following:

Equation 1 $y = 3x + 4$
Equation 2 $y = 3x - 4$

Which best describes equations 1 and 2, respectively?

1. slope of +4, y intercept of +3; slope of -4 and y intercept of -3

2. x intercept of +3, slope of +4; x intercept of -3, and slope of -4

3. y intercept of +3, slope of +4; y intercept of -3, and slope of -4

4. slope of +3, y intercept of +4; slope of +3 and y intercept of -4

196. For the following equations, solve for a and b: $30 = a + 3b - 70$ and $3a + 5b = 100$.

1. a = -50, b = 50

2. a = 5, b = -5

3. a = -5, b = 5

4. a = 50, b = -50

197. How much medicine would provide a patient with 2 tablespoons twice a day for 10 days? (1 tablespoon = 15 ml)

1. 300 ml

2. 600 ml

3. 450 ml

4. 900 ml

198. If 0.060 g of a substance is employed in preparing 125 tablets, how much substance is contained in each tablet?

    1. 390 μg

    2. 420 μg

    3. 450 μg

    4. 480 μg

199. A patient's eye patch measures 12.70 cm across. You have a tape measure in inches. How many inches does the eye patch measure? (1 in. = 2.54 cm)

    1. 17 in.

    2. 10 in.

    3. 5 in.

    4. 3 in.

200. $\left(\dfrac{1}{120} \div \dfrac{1}{150}\right) \times 50 =$

    1. $62\dfrac{1}{2}$

    2. 40

    3. $50\dfrac{1}{2}$

    4. 25

Answer Sheet
Biology

201 ① ② ③ ④   216 ① ② ③ ④   231 ① ② ③ ④   246 ① ② ③ ④   261 ① ② ③ ④

202 ① ② ③ ④   217 ① ② ③ ④   232 ① ② ③ ④   247 ① ② ③ ④   262 ① ② ③ ④

203 ① ② ③ ④   218 ① ② ③ ④   233 ① ② ③ ④   248 ① ② ③ ④   263 ① ② ③ ④

204 ① ② ③ ④   219 ① ② ③ ④   234 ① ② ③ ④   249 ① ② ③ ④   264 ① ② ③ ④

205 ① ② ③ ④   220 ① ② ③ ④   235 ① ② ③ ④   250 ① ② ③ ④   265 ① ② ③ ④

206 ① ② ③ ④   221 ① ② ③ ④   236 ① ② ③ ④   251 ① ② ③ ④   266 ① ② ③ ④

207 ① ② ③ ④   222 ① ② ③ ④   237 ① ② ③ ④   252 ① ② ③ ④   267 ① ② ③ ④

208 ① ② ③ ④   223 ① ② ③ ④   238 ① ② ③ ④   253 ① ② ③ ④   268 ① ② ③ ④

209 ① ② ③ ④   224 ① ② ③ ④   239 ① ② ③ ④   254 ① ② ③ ④   269 ① ② ③ ④

210 ① ② ③ ④   225 ① ② ③ ④   240 ① ② ③ ④   255 ① ② ③ ④   270 ① ② ③ ④

211 ① ② ③ ④   226 ① ② ③ ④   241 ① ② ③ ④   256 ① ② ③ ④   271 ① ② ③ ④

212 ① ② ③ ④   227 ① ② ③ ④   242 ① ② ③ ④   257 ① ② ③ ④   272 ① ② ③ ④

213 ① ② ③ ④   228 ① ② ③ ④   243 ① ② ③ ④   258 ① ② ③ ④   273 ① ② ③ ④

214 ① ② ③ ④   229 ① ② ③ ④   244 ① ② ③ ④   259 ① ② ③ ④   274 ① ② ③ ④

215 ① ② ③ ④   230 ① ② ③ ④   245 ① ② ③ ④   260 ① ② ③ ④   275 ① ② ③ ④

BIOLOGY

75 Questions   1 Hour 40 Minutes

Directions: Choose the best answer to each of the following questions.

201. The smallest unit of life is the

1. organ
2. organelle
3. cell
4. gene

202. The organelle primarily responsible for energy production in an aerobic cell is the

1. nucleus
2. mitochondria
3. endoplasmic reticulum
4. Golgi apparatus

203. In man, brown eyes (B) are dominant over blue eyes (b). In a cross between two Bb individuals, what percentage of offspring will have blue eyes?

1. 0%
2. 25%
3. 75%
4. 100%

204. Solutions that cause red blood cells to shrink are called

1. isotonic
2. isosmotic
3. hypertonic
4. hypotonic

205. A trace element necessary for normal health of the human body is

1. sodium
2. potassium
3. calcium
4. copper

206. Brown is the dominant color for rats, whereas white is the alternative recessive color. When a homozygous brown rat is crossed with a homozygous white rat, what percentage of the offspring is expected to be brown heterozygous?

1. 25%
2. 50%
3. 75%
4. 100%

207. Fat-soluble vitamins include all of the following except

    1. A
    2. B
    3. D
    4. K

208. Under basal conditions, the region of the body that receives the greatest blood flow is the

    1. liver
    2. brain
    3. bone
    4. skeletal muscle

209. Which of the following electrolytes is most abundant in human extracellular fluid?

    1. sodium
    2. potassium
    3. calcium
    4. magnesium

210. Most nutrients are absorbed by which region of the human gastrointestinal tract?

    1. stomach
    2. colon
    3. small intestine
    4. large intestine

211. Long-chain fatty acids normally enter the blood system in the form of

    1. cholesterol esters
    2. free fatty acids
    3. glycoproteins
    4. chylomicrons

212. The most abundant electrolyte in the intracellular fluid of man is

    1. sodium
    2. potassium
    3. calcium
    4. magnesium

213. In man, a deficiency in vitamin C (ascorbic acid) is normally associated with

    1. scurvy
    2. rickets
    3. pellagra
    4. beriberi

214. Squamous epithelium is normally associated with which region of the human body?

    1. kidney
    2. lungs
    3. skin
    4. pancreas

215. Which of the following statements is false concerning the structure of a cell?

    1. The nucleus of a cell contains DNA and is separated from the surrounding cytoplasm by a nuclear membrane.
    2. The Golgi apparatus, endoplasmic reticulum, and the majority of chromatin are found in the cytoplasm outside the nucleus.
    3. A cell with two complete sets of chromosomes is diploid.
    4. none of the above

216. Which type of muscle will contract most rapidly when stimulated?

    1. skeletal
    2. cardiac
    3. smooth
    4. All muscle types contract at the same rate.

217. Which statement about fatty acids (triglycerides) is true?

    1. Most fats containing unsaturated fatty acids are solids at room temperature, whereas fats containing saturated fatty acids are liquids.
    2. Most fatty acids in nature have an even number of carbon atoms.
    3. Fats yield approximately 50% as much energy as do carbohydrates in humans.
    4. Saturated fatty acids contain one or more double carbon bonds.

218. The nucleotide responsible for transmitting genetic information from the DNA molecule in the nucleus to the cytoplasm is

    1. transfer RNA
    2. ribosomal RNA
    3. messenger RNA
    4. none of the above

219. The proper sequence for the stages of mitosis is

    1. metaphase, prophase, anaphase, telophase
    2. prophase, anaphase, metaphase, telophase
    3. prophase, metaphase, telophase, anaphase
    4. prophase, metaphase, anaphase, telophase

220. Which statement concerning the structure and function of the biological membrane is true?

    1. Biological membranes are a sandwich composed of protein with a layer of lipid on both the inner and outer surfaces.

2. Lipid-soluble compounds tend to diffuse through biological membranes faster than water-soluble ones.
3. The rate at which lipid-soluble substances pass through biological membranes is determined by the size of the diffusing particle.
4. All of the above.

221. Passive diffusion of substances through biological membranes

1. requires energy sources such as ATP
2. causes a substance to move from a lower to a higher concentration gradient
3. can be inhibited by metabolic poisons such as cyanide
4. is a major process by which uncharged molecules can move through membranes

222. The ascending (initial) portion of an action potential observed in a cell is caused by

1. sodium influx into the cell
2. sodium efflux out of the cell
3. potassium influx into the cell
4. potassium efflux out of the cell

223. The descending portion of an action potential after the initial spike potential in a cell is caused by

1. sodium influx into the cell
2. sodium efflux out of the cell
3. potassium influx into the cell
4. potassium efflux out of the cell

224. The normal resting potential of the inner side of a nerve cell relative to the outer side is

1. 100 mV
2. 50 mV
3. -50 mV
4. -500 mV

225. Which of the following endogenous substances does not actively aid in the digestion of dietary nutrients?

1. pepsin
2. insulin
3. lactase
4. trypsin

226. The organ primarily responsible for detoxifying toxic substances in the blood is the

1. lung
2. kidney
3. liver
4. pancreas

227. In man, the removal of waste products from the blood is one of the primary functions of the

    1. liver
    2. pancreas
    3. kidneys
    4. spleen

228. Absorption of dietary nutrients can be accomplished by which process?

    1. active transport
    2. facilitated diffusion
    3. passive diffusion
    4. all of the above

229. In humans, bile salts play an important role in enhancing the intestinal absorption of

    1. fatty acids
    2. glucose
    3. thiamine
    4. amino acids

230. Which of the following sugars is not classified as a simple sugar that can be directly absorbed from the digestive tract in man?

    1. glucose
    2. fructose
    3. glycogen
    4. galactose

231. Which organ of the human body is first affected by a rapid decrease of glucose concentration in the blood?

    1. brain
    2. heart
    3. kidneys
    4. eyes

232. In man, night blindness can be due to a diet deficient in

    1. iron
    2. copper
    3. vitamin K
    4. vitamin A

233. The transport process that does not require the presence of a carrier is

    1. active transport
    2. passive diffusion
    3. facilitated diffusion
    4. none of the above

234. Saturation kinetics are not usually observed in which of the following transport processes?

    1. active transport
    2. passive diffusion
    3. facilitated diffusion
    4. phagocytosis

235. Which theory states that genes exist in individuals as pairs?

    1. the theory of recapitulation
    2. Starling's law
    3. Mendel's law of segregation
    4. the Watson-Crick model

236. Of the following, the element least abundant in the human body is

    1. carbon
    2. oxygen
    3. hydrogen
    4. calcium

237. Each cell of every organism of a given species contains a characteristic number of chromosomes. How many chromosomes are found in each cell of the human body?

    1. 13
    2. 23
    3. 46
    4. 48

238. In man, which blood type is known as the universal donor?

    1. O negative
    2. O positive
    3. AB negative
    4. AB positive

239. All of the following substances are known to be neurotransmitters at neuromuscular junctions except

    1. epinephrine
    2. norepinephrine
    3. acetylcholine
    4. cholecystokinin

240. Certain white blood cells are produced in lymphoid tissue such as the spleen, thymus, and lymph nodes. Which of the following white blood cells is produced by lymphoid tissue?

    1. neutrophils
    2. monocytes
    3. eosinophils
    4. none of the above

241. Immunity produced in response to vaccination with some foreign protein (antigen) is known as

    1. actively acquired immunity
    2. passively acquired immunity
    3. natural immunity
    4. cellular immunity

242. The major process by which the kidney removes waste products from the blood is called

    1. tubular secretion
    2. tubular reabsorption
    3. glomerular filtration
    4. tubular sublimation

243. Stimulation of the human sympathetic nervous system causes all of the following changes in the body except

    1. increased heart rate
    2. increased sweating
    3. constriction of pupils
    4. increased blood pressure

244. Fatigue of a muscle that has contracted many times is primarily caused by an accumulation of

    1. carbon dioxide
    2. lactic acid
    3. urea
    4. sodium chloride

245. Cell division during which the chromosome number is reduced from diploid to haploid is known as

    1. mitosis
    2. synapsis
    3. meiosis
    4. karyokinesis

246. The appearance of any individual with respect to a given inherited trait is known as its

    1. genotype
    2. phenotype
    3. recessive trait
    4. heterozygous trait

247. Which of the following disease states is known to be caused by homozygous recessive genes in an individual?

    1. sickle cell anemia
    2. beriberi
    3. hypertension
    4. pellagra

248. Intense exercise and training of an athlete can result in which of the following changes?

    1. increase in the number of muscle fibers
    2. increased respiratory rate
    3. increase in the size of muscle fibers
    4. both 1 and 3

249. During sperm formation, spermatids

    1. develop directly from primary spermatocytes
    2. contain the diploid number of chromosomes
    3. develop immediately after the first meiotic division
    4. develop immediately after the second meiotic division

250. An individual with type A negative blood can receive blood from which of the following blood types?

    1. O negative
    2. A positive
    3. O positive
    4. all of the above

251. Vestigial organs are the remnants of organs that were functional in some ancestral animal. In man, which organ(s) is not vestigial in nature?

    1. appendix
    2. wisdom teeth
    3. coccygeal vertebrae
    4. pupils of the eyes

252. Which of the following graphs most accurately shows the relation between the substrate (S) and product (P) in a saturated irreversible enzymatic reaction?

1.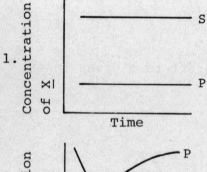

2.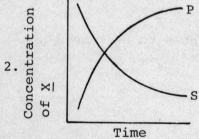

3.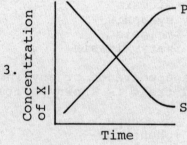

4.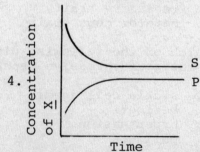

253. Oxygen and carbon dioxide are primarily transported through the blood

    1. dissolved in plasma water
    2. bound to plasma proteins
    3. bound to hemoglobin
    4. none of the above

254. Which of the following statements is false concerning the genetics of man and animals?

    1. Inbreeding is harmful and leads to the production of genetically inferior offspring.
    2. Defective traits can be sex linked.
    3. Outbreeding is the mating of two totally unrelated individuals.
    4. Vigorous inbreeding can result in a high frequency of defects present at birth termed congenital anomalies.

255. Which of the following graphs most accurately shows the relationship between the substrate (S) and product (P) in a reversible unsaturated enzymatic reaction?

1.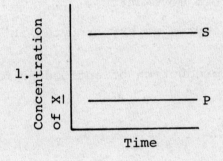

2.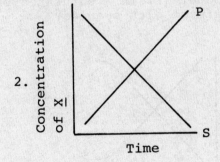

3.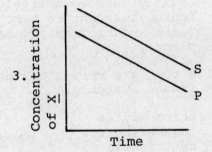

4.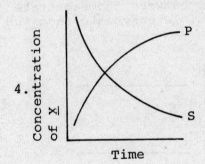

256. The members of two different species of animals or plants that share the same living space or food source may interact with each other in a positive or negative manner. Which of the following would be a negative interaction?

    1. parasitism
    2. commensalism
    3. protocooperation
    4. mutualism

257. Which of the following plasma proteins is most responsible for the colloid osmotic pressure that regulates the water content of the plasma?

    1. fibrinogen
    2. albumin
    3. hemoglobin
    4. gammaglobulin

258. Which of the following statements is false concerning leukocytes in the human body?

    1. Leukocytes are white blood cells.
    2. Leukocytes move actively by amoeboid movement.
    3. Leukocytes contain hemoglobin.
    4. There are the same number of leukocytes as erythrocytes in plasma.

259. Cells that are very important in the production of antibodies for the immune system are

    1. thrombocytes
    2. megakaryocytes
    3. neutrophils
    4. plasma cells

260. Which of the following graphs most accurately shows the relationship between the substrate (S) and product (P) in a saturated reversible enzymatic reaction after treatment with cyanide?

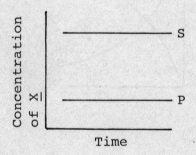 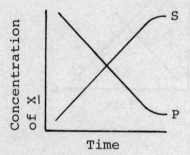

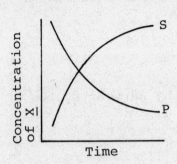

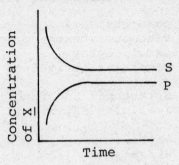

261. The transport of oxygen and carbon dioxide in the blood depends largely on which component of the red blood cell?

    1. cell wall
    2. nucleus
    3. hemoglobin
    4. cytoplasm

262. The plasma protein most abundant in plasma is

    1. albumin
    2. globulin
    3. fibrinogen
    4. immunoglobin

263. Which of the following conditions does not increase the number of red blood cells in the human body?

    1. high altitude environment
    2. low oxygen delivery to the tissues
    3. increased erythropoietin production
    4. increased carbon dioxide concentration in the blood

264. Which of the following is not associated with heat loss in man?

    1. sweating
    2. increased muscle tone
    3. decreased metabolism
    4. vasodilation

265. Substances that are actively reabsorbed by the kidney tubules include

    1. urea
    2. creatinine
    3. glucose
    4. all of the above

266. Tissues of the body that are normally involved in regulating the volume of body fluids do not include

    1. baroreceptors
    2. vasomotor center of the brain
    3. osmoreceptor
    4. reticular activating system

267. The structural and functional unit of the nervous system of all multicellular animals is the

    1. axon
    2. nerve
    3. neuron
    4. dendrite

268. Which of the following statements about the rate of conduction for a nerve impulse is true in man?

    1. The rate of conduction increases as the diameter of the axon increases.
    2. The rate of conduction is faster in smaller nerve fibers than in larger ones.
    3. Myelin sheaths usually decrease the rate of conduction.
    4. all of the above

269. Which of the following statements concerning the human autonomic nervous system is true?

    1. It controls the voluntary movements of muscles in the limbs.
    2. It is composed of both sympathetic and parasympathetic nerves.
    3. Motor impulses reach the effector organ from the brain or spinal cord by a single neuron.
    4. all of the above.

270. In man, hormones that are derived from amino acids include

    1. prostaglandins
    2. estradiol
    3. testosterone
    4. thyroxine

271. When a skeletal muscle fiber is given a single stimulus, a single twitch with numerous electrical phases is observed. What is the correct order for the phases or periods seen in a skeletal muscle fiber after stimulation?

    1. contraction, latent, relaxation, refractory
    2. refractory, contraction, latent, relaxation
    3. latent, contraction, relaxation, refractory
    4. latent, refractory, contraction, relaxation

272. Which statement is false concerning the role of hormones in the human body?

    1. Hormones can be secreted by one part of the body, pass through the blood, and act on a target organ in another part of the body.
    2. Neurohormones may pass down axons to the target organ in another part of the body.
    3. Hormones can be derivatives of amino acids, fatty acids, or long peptides.
    4. Hormones usually provide instantaneous control of a bodily function.

273. Hormones for the regulation of the menstrual cycle in women include

    1. progesterone
    2. vasopressin
    3. aldosterone
    4. none of the above

274. In the human eye, the rods located in the retina are responsible for

    1. color vision
    2. bright light vision
    3. peripheral vision
    4. all of the above

275. Which of the following statements is not true in reference to the human lymphatic system?

    1. The rate of lymph flow is similar to that of the circulation.
    2. The lymphatic system is an auxiliary system for return of fluid from the tissue spaces to the circulation.
    3. Lymph nodes produce one type of white blood cells, known as lymphocytes.
    4. The lymphatic system plays an important role in the immune process.

Answer Sheet
Chemistry

276 ① ② ③ ④	296 ① ② ③ ④	316 ① ② ③ ④	336 ① ② ③ ④	356 ① ② ③ ④
277 ① ② ③ ④	297 ① ② ③ ④	317 ① ② ③ ④	337 ① ② ③ ④	357 ① ② ③ ④
278 ① ② ③ ④	298 ① ② ③ ④	318 ① ② ③ ④	338 ① ② ③ ④	358 ① ② ③ ④
279 ① ② ③ ④	299 ① ② ③ ④	319 ① ② ③ ④	339 ① ② ③ ④	359 ① ② ③ ④
280 ① ② ③ ④	300 ① ② ③ ④	320 ① ② ③ ④	340 ① ② ③ ④	360 ① ② ③ ④
281 ① ② ③ ④	301 ① ② ③ ④	321 ① ② ③ ④	341 ① ② ③ ④	361 ① ② ③ ④
282 ① ② ③ ④	302 ① ② ③ ④	322 ① ② ③ ④	342 ① ② ③ ④	362 ① ② ③ ④
283 ① ② ③ ④	303 ① ② ③ ④	323 ① ② ③ ④	343 ① ② ③ ④	363 ① ② ③ ④
284 ① ② ③ ④	304 ① ② ③ ④	324 ① ② ③ ④	344 ① ② ③ ④	364 ① ② ③ ④
285 ① ② ③ ④	305 ① ② ③ ④	325 ① ② ③ ④	345 ① ② ③ ④	365 ① ② ③ ④
286 ① ② ③ ④	306 ① ② ③ ④	326 ① ② ③ ④	346 ① ② ③ ④	366 ① ② ③ ④
287 ① ② ③ ④	307 ① ② ③ ④	327 ① ② ③ ④	347 ① ② ③ ④	367 ① ② ③ ④
288 ① ② ③ ④	308 ① ② ③ ④	328 ① ② ③ ④	348 ① ② ③ ④	368 ① ② ③ ④
289 ① ② ③ ④	309 ① ② ③ ④	329 ① ② ③ ④	349 ① ② ③ ④	369 ① ② ③ ④
290 ① ② ③ ④	310 ① ② ③ ④	330 ① ② ③ ④	350 ① ② ③ ④	370 ① ② ③ ④
291 ① ② ③ ④	311 ① ② ③ ④	331 ① ② ③ ④	351 ① ② ③ ④	371 ① ② ③ ④
292 ① ② ③ ④	312 ① ② ③ ④	332 ① ② ③ ④	352 ① ② ③ ④	372 ① ② ③ ④
293 ① ② ③ ④	313 ① ② ③ ④	333 ① ② ③ ④	353 ① ② ③ ④	373 ① ② ③ ④
294 ① ② ③ ④	314 ① ② ③ ④	334 ① ② ③ ④	354 ① ② ③ ④	374 ① ② ③ ④
295 ① ② ③ ④	315 ① ② ③ ④	335 ① ② ③ ④	355 ① ② ③ ④	375 ① ② ③ ④

CHEMISTRY

100 Questions   2 Hours

Directions: Choose the best answer to each of the following questions.

276. Alkanes are not

1. saturated compounds containing carbon and hydrogen

2. formed from $\underline{sp}^3$ hybrid orbitals

3. arranged in a straight-chain sequence

4. of the general formula $C_{\underline{n}}H_{2\underline{n}}$

277. Regarding phenol,

1. a nitro substituent in the ortho position will lower the $\underline{K_a}$

2. a methyl substituent in the ortho position will lower the $\underline{K_a}$

3. a methyl substituent in the ortho position will increase the $\underline{K_a}$

4. the OH substituent is a meta-directing group

278. Which of the following is false?

1. $pH = \dfrac{(\log(1}{[H^+])}$

2. $pH + pOH = 14$

3. $(H^+)(OH^-) = 10^{-14}$

4. $pH - pOH = 14$

279. Calculate the percentage of iron in hematite (Fe_2O_3), given the atomic weights of Fe = 56 and O = 16.

1. 70%

2. 2%

3. 30%

4. 49%

280. How many liters of hydrogen are required to produce 20 liters of ammonia, given the equation $3H_2 + N_2 \longrightarrow 2NH_3$?

1. 15 liters

2. 30 liters

3. $33\frac{1}{3}$ liters

4. 40 liters

281. The volume occupied by the gram-molecular weight of a gas at 0°C and 760 mmHg is

1. 1 liter

2. 22.4 liters

3. 32 liters

4. 100 liters

282. Given the atomic weights of C = 12 and O = 16, what is the weight of 2 liters of carbon dioxide at standard temperature and pressure?

1. 2 g

2. 4 g

3. 6 g

4. 8 g

283. Which of the following hybrid orbitals would carbon form in acetylene?

1. sp

2. sp^2

3. sp^3

4. all of the above

284. Which of the following hybrid orbitals would methane and water both form?

1. sp

2. sp^2

3. sp^3

4. all of the above

285. The structural formula indicates all of the following except

1. the number of atoms in a molecule

2. the gram-molecular volume

3. the types of atoms present

4. the arrangement of the atom

286. Pick out the wrong statement.

1. Organic compounds may exist as isomers.

2. Reactions involving organic compounds always proceed faster than those involving inorganic compounds.

3. Organic compounds are generally soluble in organic solvents.

4. Organic compounds decompose at relatively lower temperatures than inorganic compounds.

287. When the nucleus of an atom emits a beta particle,

1. the atomic weight decreases by 4

2. the atomic weight increases by 1

3. the atomic number increases by 1

4. the atomic number stays the same

288. The conversion of one element into another is termed

1. transformation

2. disintegration

3. transmutation

4. emanation

289. All the following are characteristics of gamma rays except

1. high-energy x rays

2. very short wavelength

3. deflected by electric fields

4. travel at the speed of light

290. The energy released in nuclear reactions is due to

1. atomic fusion

2. electron capture

3. atomic fission

4. both fusion and fission

291. All of the following are alcohols except

1. methanol

2. ethanol

3. glycerine

4. sodium hydroxide

292. Pick out the incorrect statement concerning hydrogen chloride gas.

1. It is lighter than air.

2. It has a pungent smell.

3. It is soluble in water.

4. It reacts with ammonia-forming ammonium chloride.

293. The following are halogens except

1. bromine

2. iodine

3. chlorine

4. turpentine

294. The number of equivalents per mole for $HC_2H_3O_2$ is

1. 1

2. 2

3. 3

4. 4

295. Avogadro's law states that

1. under identical temperature and pressure, only certain gases contain the same number of molecules

2. all gases contain different numbers of molecules, irrespective of pressure or temperature conditions

3. only under equal volumes will all gases contain the same number of molecules

4. under identical conditions of temperature and pressure, equal volumes of all gases contain the same number of molecules

296. The volume of a sample of gas was 300 ml at 27°C and 380 mmHg. What is its volume at standard conditions of temperature and pressure?

    1. 116.0 ml

    2. 126.0 ml

    3. 136.0 ml

    4. 22.4 ml

297. According to the equation $Fe + I_2 = FeI_2$, how much iodine is needed to react with 10 g of iron? (Fe = 56, I = 127).

    1. 45 g

    2. 55 g

    3. 35 g

    4. 65 g

298. Calculate the amount of sodium chloride crystals needed to supply 100 mg of sodium ions (Na = 23, Cl = 35.5).

    1. 180 mg

    2. 432 mg

    3. 355 mg

    4. 254 mg

299. Now calculate the concentration (in milligrams per milliliter) of a solution containing 2 mEq of sodium chloride per milliliter.

    1. 585 mg/ml

    2. 355 mg/ml

    3. 230 mg/ml

    4. 117 mg/ml

300. It has been ordered that Mr. Smith should receive 2 mEq of sodium chloride per kilogram of body weight. Since Mr. Smith weighs 60 kg, how much sodium chloride is needed?

1. 7 g

2. 17 g

3. 27 g

4. 117 g

301. Since the hospital stocks a 0.9% solution of sodium chloride, how much of this solution must be administered to Mr. Smith?

1. 777 ml

2. 350 ml

3. 3500 ml

4. 7700 ml

302. The pharmacy, however, could only supply a 0.45% solution of sodium chloride. How many liters of this solution must be given to Mr. Smith?

1. 1.5 liters

2. 3.0 liters

3. 4.5 liters

4. 6.0 liters

303. Electrolytes (e.g., sodium chloride) are important in establishing osmotic pressure; the unit used in measuring osmotic activity is the milliosmol. How many milliosmols of particles does 1 mmole of sodium chloride present?

1. 1 mOsm

2. 2 mOsm

3. 3 mOsm

4. none of the above

304. Osmotic activity is a function of

1. electrolytes only

2. nonelectrolytes only

3. strong electrolytes only

4. the total number of particles present in solution

305. If one assumes complete dissociation, how many milliosmols of sodium chloride are in 100 ml of a 0.9% solution?

    1. 2 mOsm

    2. 3 mOsm

    3. 31 mOsm

    4. 45 mOsm

306. Pick out the false statement.

    1. Hydrogen has one proton.

    2. Hydrogen has one electron in the K shell.

    3. Hydrogen has one neutron in its nucleus.

    4. Hydrogen has an atomic number and an atomic weight of 1.

307. Beryllium has five neutrons and two electrons each in the K and L shells, respectively. Therefore beryllium has

    1. an atomic weight of 5 and an atomic number of 4

    2. an atomic weight of 9 and an atomic number of 5

    3. an atomic weight of 4 and an atomic number of 9

    4. an atomic weight of 9 and an atomic number of 4

308. The chemical symbol for mercury is Hg, whereas that for oxygen is O. If HgO is mercuric oxide, what is mercurous oxide?

    1. HgO_2

    2. Hg_2O

    3. Hg_2O_3

    4. Hg_3O_2

309. HNO_3 is the chemical formula for nitric acid; HNO_2 is the chemical formula for

    1. nitrous acid

    2. nitronous acid

    3. nitrate acid

    4. nitrite acid

310. The combination of an element A with an element B to form a new compound AB is called a synthetic reaction. The reverse of this reaction is called

    1. single replacement

    2. synthesis

    3. decomposition

    4. double replacement

311. Pick out the incorrect statement.

    1. Oxidation is associated with the loss of electrons.

    2. Oxidation-reduction reactions involve the loss and gain of electrons.

    3. The oxidized particle (atom) shows a decrease in valence number.

    4. Reduction involves the gain of electrons.

312. You are given the equation $ABC_3 \longrightarrow AB + C_2$. The balanced equation is

    1. $2ABC_3 \longrightarrow AB + 3C_2$

    2. $ABC_3 \longrightarrow AB + C_2$

    3. $2ABC_3 \longrightarrow 2AB + 3C_2$

    4. $3ABC_3 \longrightarrow 3AB + 3C_2$

313. A molecule of oxygen contains two atoms of oxygen. How many atoms of oxygen does a molecule of ozone contain?

    1. two

    2. four

    3. one

    4. three

314. Which statement is false?

    1. Oxygen burns by itself.

    2. Oxygen is an odorless and colorless gas.

    3. Oxygen supports combustion.

4. Air contains about 20% oxygen.

315. Hydrogen peroxide decomposes to yield

1. two molecules of water and two molecules of oxygen

2. one molecule of water and one molecule of oxygen

3. three molecules of water and two molecules of oxygen

4. two molecules of water and one molecule of oxygen

316. A volumetric flask contains 5000 ml of water. What is the weight of this quantity of water?

1. 50 g

2. 500 g

3. 5000 g

4. 50,000 g

317. Molarity ($\underline{M}$) is best defined as

1. moles of solute per kiloliter of solution

2. moles of solute per kilogram of solution

3. moles of solute per 100 ml of solution

4. moles of solute per liter of solution

318. A total of 40 g of sodium hydroxide is dissolved in water to give a final volume of 400 ml. What is the molarity of this solution? (Na = 23, O = 16, H = 1)

1. 0.25 $\underline{M}$

2. 2.5 $\underline{M}$

3. 25 $\underline{M}$

4. 0.1 $\underline{M}$

319. How many moles of solute are there in 125 ml of a 5 $\underline{M}$ solution of sodium hydroxide?

1. 10.0 mol

2. 3.40 mol

3. 0.625 mol

4. 6.25 mol

320. Now, how much sodium hydroxide is there in 125 ml of a 5 $\underline{M}$ solution of sodium hydroxide?

1. 75.0 g

2. 62.5 g

3. 25.0 g

4. 80.5 g

321. What is the molarity of 1 liter of pure water (H_2O)?

1. 55 $\underline{M}$

2. 18 $\underline{M}$

3. 19 $\underline{M}$

4. cannot be determined

322. All of the following are colligative properties of solutions except

1. the boiling point

2. the vapor pressure

3. the freezing point

4. the specific gravity

323. Given that the hydrogen ion concentration (moles per liter) of a solution is 1.0, what is its pH?

1. 0

2. 1

3. 7

4. 14

324. Given the same hydrogen ion concentration (in moles/liter) of 1.0, calculate the pH value of this solution.

1. 0

2. 1

3. 7

4. 14

325. The higher the pH of a solution

1. the lower the acidity

2. the higher the hydrogen ion concentration

3. the lower the basicity

4. the stronger the acid

326. Pick out the false statement.

1. Methane is important in addition reactions.

2. Methane is explosive when combined with air.

3. Methane is a major component of natural gas.

4. Methane is commonly known as marsh gas.

327. All of the following are esters except

1. ethyl acetate

2. methyl salicylate

3. sodium formate

4. nitroglycerine

328. Carbohydrates are compounds containing carbon, hydrogen, and oxygen. Which of the following is not a carbohydrate?

1. glucose

2. glyceryl stearate

3. dextran

4. cellulose

329. Pick out the nonsynthetic fiber.

1. cellulose

2. rayon

3. Orlon

4. nylon

330. The uncertainty principle, which states that it is impossible to know with exactitude both the momentum and position of an electron simultaneously, is associated with

1. Heisenberg

2. Planck

3. de Broglie

4. Bohr

331. How many quantum numbers are necessary in order to define electronic wave functions?

1. 4

2. 3

3. 2

4. 1

332. Wolfgang Pauli's exclusion principle states that

1. no two electrons in an atom can have the same three quantum numbers

2. no two electrons in an atom can have the same four quantum numbers

3. no two electrons can have the same orbital

4. any two electrons in an atom can have the same four quantum numbers

333. The electronic distribution in the orbitals of an oxygen atom is

1. $1s^2 2s^4 2p^2$

2. $1s^2 2s^2 2p^4$

3. $1s^2 2s^2 2p^8$

4. $1s^2 2s^2 2p^6$

334. Carbon has six protons and its atomic weight is 12. How many electrons and neutrons does it have?

1. 3 electrons, 9 neutrons

2. 6 electrons, 6 neutrons

3. 6 electrons, 12 neutrons

4. cannot be determined from the information given

335. Name the element with the electronic distribution $1s^2 2s^2 2p^2$.

    1. helium

    2. carbon

    3. beryllium

    4. oxygen

336. Isotopes are atoms of elements differing only in

    1. valence

    2. the number of electrons

    3. chemical property

    4. mass

337. Carbon-14 is a commonly used radioisotope in medical research. How many more neutrons does it have compared to natural carbon?

    1. 2

    2. 4

    3. 6

    4. 0

338. Pick out the statement about gamma-ray decay that is false.

    1. The number of protons does not change.

    2. It results in a decrease of 4 units of atomic mass.

    3. There is emission of photons.

    4. The number of neutrons does not change.

339. Electromagnetic radiation has a wide spectrum of energies and wavelengths. The angstrom is widely used as a unit to measure wavelength. What does it equal in meters?

1. 1×10^{-15} m

2. 1×10^{-9} m

3. 1×10^{-10} m

4. 1×10^{-11} m

340. Pyrophosphoric acid is $H_4P_2O_7$. What does the prefix <u>pyro</u> indicate?

   1. lowest oxidation state

   2. highest oxidation state

   3. highest hydrated form

   4. loss of water

341. Lead (Pb) has many industrial uses. Lead ion exists in two oxidation states, which are

   1. divalent and tetravalent

   2. monovalent and trivalent

   3. divalent and pentavalent

   4. monovalent and divalent

342. Plaster of Paris is made by heating gypsum until it loses three-fourths of its water of hydration. What alkaline-earth metal is found in gypsum and plaster of Paris?

   1. phosphorus

   2. calcium

   3. magnesium

   4. barium

343. Hydrogen sulfide (H_2S) can be prepared by the action of an acid on any metallic sulfide. All of the following are characteristics of hydrogen sulfide except

   1. colorless gas

   2. denser than air

   3. non-toxic

   4. odor of rotten eggs

344. What is the common name for the organic acid with the formula CH_3COOH?

    1. aqua fortis

    2. muriatic acid

    3. aqua regia

    4. vinegar

345. If table salt is sodium chloride, give the formula for baking soda.

    1. $Na_2B_4O_7$

    2. $MgSO_4$

    3. Na_2CO_3

    4. $NaHCO_3$

346. HOCl is a more powerful oxidizing agent than chlorine. What is HOCl?

    1. tincture of iodine

    2. chloroform

    3. hypochlorous acid

    4. brine

347. Alkenes do not possess

    1. a pi bond

    2. an alpha bond

    3. a double bond

    4. a sigma bond

348. Amino acids are generally represented by the formula RNH_2COOH. What class of organic compounds is represented by $RCONH_2$?

    1. amides

    2. esters

    3. amines

    4. azides

349. In chemistry, the suffix ase, as in lipase, denotes

1. a carboxyl group

2. a base

3. an enzyme

4. a sugar

350. A primary alcohol has at least two hydrogens attached to the alcohol carbon. A tertiary alcohol has

1. no hydrogens attached to the alcohol carbon

2. only hydrogen attached to the alcohol carbon

3. three hydrogens attached to the alcohol carbon

4. only one hydrogen attached to the alcohol carbon

351. Which of the formulas below is methyl vinyl ketone?

1. $CH_3OCH_2CH=CH_2$

2. $CH_3COCH=CH_2$

3. $CH_3CH_2CH_2=COOH$

4. $CH_3CH_2COCH=CH_2$

352. The incorrect way of naming an organic acid is

1. by using the hydrocarbon name of the longest chain

2. by designating the carboxyl carbon as carbon number 1

3. by changing the suffix from ane to anoic

4. by changing the suffix from ane to ol

353. Name the hydrocarbon, $CH_3(CH_2)_8CH_3$.

1. nonane

2. octane

3. undecane

4. decane

354. Pick out the incorrect statement.

   1. Atoms connected by single bonds rotate around the bond.

   2. Atoms in double bonds are not free to rotate.

   3. Atoms in a ring are free to rotate around their bonds.

   4. Atoms in triple bonds are not free to rotate.

355. Pick out the incorrect statement.

   1. The stability of a carbonium ion is increased by charge dispersal.

   2. A primary carbonium ion forms more easily than a tertiary carbonium ion.

   3. The carbon atom in a carbonium ion has only six electrons.

   4. Carbonium ions can be classified as primary, secondary, or tertiary.

356. With regard to benzene, one of the following statements is incorrect.

   1. It is a flat (planar) molecule.

   2. It has the formula C_6H_6.

   3. It is a symmetrical molecule.

   4. It has a bond angle of 150°.

357. With regard to the carbonyl carbons of aldehydes and ketones, one of the following statements is false.

   1. They usually have a bond angle of 120°.

   2. They are oriented such that carbon and oxygen are joined by a double bond.

   3. They are $\underline{sp}^2$ hybridized and not planar.

   4. They are connected to three other atoms by sigma bonds.

358. Nucleophilic substitution is commonly encountered in organic chemistry. Only one statement below is correct, concerning nucleophilic displacement.

   1. Amines are more reactive than amides.

   2. Acid chlorides are more reactive than alkyl chloride.

3. Ethers are more reactive than esters.

4. Saturated carbons are more reactive than acyl carbon.

359. Glycols are

1. alcohols containing two hydroxyl groups

2. alcohols without any hydroxyl group

3. aldehydes containing two hydroxyl groups

4. ketones containing two hydroxyl groups

360. The Grignard reagent is very useful in organic chemistry. Pick out the one incorrect statement about it.

1. Its general name is alkylmagnesium halide.

2. The magnesium-halogen bond is covalent.

3. The carbon-magnesium bond is considered covalent.

4. Its general formula is RMgX.

361. Which is the correct statement?

1. Optically inactive reactants yield optically active products.

2. Optically active products are the result of optically inactive reactants.

3. Optically inactive reactants yield optically inactive products.

4. The preparation of dissymmetric compounds from symmetric reactants yields no racemic modification.

362. If CH_4 is methane, what is CH_2?

1. methanol

2. mesyl

3. methyl

4. methylene

363. The Diels-Alder reaction does not involve

1. a diene and a dienophile

2. a product that is six membered

3. α β -unsaturated carbonyl compounds

4. electron-releasing groups in the dienophile

364. Disaccharides are composed of two monosaccharide units. Which of the following is not a disaccharide?

1. amylose

2. lactose

3. maltose

4. sucrose

365. Which of the following amino acids is simplest in structure?

1. arginine

2. tyrosine

3. glycine

4. methionine

366. Aryl halides are compounds containing

1. halogen attached to a side chain of an aromatic ring

2. halogen attached directly to an aromatic ring

3. halogen attached directly to a cyclic alkane

4. halogen attached to an alkene

367. Ethylene oxide is best described as

1. an alkane

2. an alkene

3. an aldehyde

4. an epoxide

368. Amines may have all of the following formulas except

1. RNH_2

2. R_3N

3. RNH

4. R_2NH

369. Absolute alcohol is

    1. a mixture of 50 parts of alcohol to water

    2. 80% alcohol

    3. water-free alcohol

    4. wood alcohol

370. Two aromatic rings sharing a pair of carbon atoms are called fused-ring hydrocarbons. The simplest member of this family of compounds is

    1. naphthalene

    2. phenanthrene

    3. benzene

    4. anthracene

371. CH_3OH is usually known as

    1. menthone

    2. methanol

    3. menthol

    4. mesitol

372. All the following describes Tollen's reagent except

    1. reduction of silver ion to free silver

    2. oxidation of an aldehyde

    3. reduction of an acid to aldehyde

    4. silver ammonia ion

373. In forming ammonia, nitrogen uses

    1. $\underline{sp}$ orbitals

    2. $\underline{sp}^1$ orbitals

    3. $\underline{sp}^2$ orbitals

    4. $\underline{sp}^3$ orbitals

374. An acid chloride can be prepared by substitution of the hydroxyl group of a carboxylic acid. The following reagents are commonly used to prepare acid chlorides except

1. thionyl chloride

2. ethyl chloride

3. phosphorus trichloride

4. phosphorus pentachloride

375. Which is the incorrect statement?

1. Sucrose is a reducing sugar.

2. All monosaccharides are reducing sugars.

3. Glucose is a monosaccharide.

4. Glucose is a reducing sugar.

Answer Sheet
Reading Comprehension

376 ① ② ③ ④   385 ① ② ③ ④   394 ① ② ③ ④   403 ① ② ③ ④   412 ① ② ③ ④

377 ① ② ③ ④   386 ① ② ③ ④   395 ① ② ③ ④   404 ① ② ③ ④   413 ① ② ③ ④

378 ① ② ③ ④   387 ① ② ③ ④   396 ① ② ③ ④   405 ① ② ③ ④   414 ① ② ③ ④

379 ① ② ③ ④   388 ① ② ③ ④   397 ① ② ③ ④   406 ① ② ③ ④   415 ① ② ③ ④

380 ① ② ③ ④   389 ① ② ③ ④   398 ① ② ③ ④   407 ① ② ③ ④   416 ① ② ③ ④

381 ① ② ③ ④   390 ① ② ③ ④   399 ① ② ③ ④   408 ① ② ③ ④   417 ① ② ③ ④

382 ① ② ③ ④   391 ① ② ③ ④   400 ① ② ③ ④   409 ① ② ③ ④   418 ① ② ③ ④

383 ① ② ③ ④   392 ① ② ③ ④   401 ① ② ③ ④   410 ① ② ③ ④

384 ① ② ③ ④   393 ① ② ③ ④   402 ① ② ③ ④   411 ① ② ③ ④

READING COMPREHENSION

43 Questions   45 Minutes

Directions: Read each of the following passages and choose the best answer to the questions that follow each passage.

1   Before the intravenous administration of a medication, it is essential to check the medication, dose, fluid in which the drug is to be given, and time of administration against the patient's chart. After this, all the necessary
5   equipment, such as an alcohol or iodophor sponge, a needle an intravenous board, tape, and the intravenous solution or admixture, should be assembled. The patient should then be identified by his armband and the procedure explained to the patient to alleviate any apprehension. Venipuncture can then
10   be performed using a needle or catheter that should be checked after insertion to ensure that it is properly placed in the vein and adequately secured to the patient's arm. The patient should be advised not to disturb the venipuncture site. Because the rate of flow of the solution can be affected by nu-
15   merous variables (gravity, solution viscosity, temperature, and possibly defective equipment), it should be checked every hour or so, depending on hospital policy. When the rate of flow is critical, such as in pediatric patients or in paren-teral nutrition, an infusion pump may be needed to ensure the
20   proper flow of solution into the patient.

376. Which of the following items is not part of the necessary equipment for administering an intravenous medication?

    1. alcohol sponge or swab
    2. needle
    3. intravenous solution
    4. intramuscular solution

377. Which of the following is a variable that affects the rate of flow of medication?

    1. solution color
    2. solution viscosity
    3. solution smell
    4. solution particle size

378. On what kinds of patients should an infusion pump be used?

    1. pediatric patients
    2. adult patients
    3. geriatric patients
    4. comatose patients

379. Which of the following must one check before administering an in-
      travenous solution?

       1. the time
       2. the medication against the chart
       3. the day
       4. the dose of the intramuscular drug

1   Adrenergic agents, commonly found in appetite suppres-
          sants, bronchodilators, central nervous system stimulants,
          and vasoconstrictors, produce slight pupillary dilation.
          They have not been observed to produce any adverse effects
5   in open-angle glaucoma, and the incidence of deleterious ef-
          fects on angle closure glaucoma after systemic administration
          has been extremely low. Adrenergic agents such as epinephrine
          and phenylephrine have been used ocularly to treat open-
          angle glaucoma. It is important to note, however, that these
10   agents will elevate the intraocular pressure by narrowing the
          anterior chamber angle when instilled into eyes of angle clo-
          sure patients.

                  General anesthetics producing parasympathetic and sym-
          pathetic imbalance may cause pupillary block. To prevent this
15   complication, topical pilocarpine at 1% may be instilled into
          the eye 1 hr prior to anesthesia.

380. Adrenergic agents are commonly found in all of the following ex-
      cept

       1. bronchodilators
       2. bronchoconstrictors
       3. vasoconstrictors
       4. appetite suppressants

381. General anesthetics that produce parasympathetic and sympathetic
      imbalance may cause

       1. pupillary constriction
       2. pupillary dilation
       3. pupillary block
       4. pupillary stimulation

382. Adrenergic agents may cause _____ in intraocular pressure.

       1. a decrease
       2. an increase
       3. a slight change
       4. no change

383. Which adrenergic agents have been used to treat open-angle glau-
      coma?

       1. epinephrine and ACTH
       2. epinephrine and propranolol
       3. epinephrine and phenylephrine
       4. epinephrine and droperidol

384. Pilocarpine administered _____ hour(s) before anesthesia can prevent the pupillary block caused by anesthetics.

    1. 4
    2. 2
    3. 1½
    4. 1

1   There are numerous methods of administering diphenylhydantoin; however, the regimen must be prescribed individually
for each patient because of the many variables that influence
the absorption, distribution, metabolism, and excretion of
5   diphenylhydantoin. Ventricular tachycardia usually requires
intravenous therapy. There appears to be no indication in
this situation for intramuscular injections, because the drug
is slowly and erratically absorbed from the site, besides being very painful. Diphenylhydantoin plasma levels after in-
10 tramuscular injection may be 25-50% lower than after equivalent
oral doses. Doses of 50-100 mg of diphenylhydantoin, up to
a maximum of 1.0 g, may be administered intravenously every
5 min, producing only a mild decrease (10-30 mmHg) in sys-
tolic blood pressure. Single intravenous doses of 300 mg
15 or more produce a more marked hypotension (20-45 mmHg) and
also lead to subtherapeutic diphenylhydantoin plasma levels
within 20-40 minutes. Generally, cardiovascular complications
can be avoided with an infusion rate of 20-50 mg/min.

385. Treatment of ventricular tachycardia with diphenylhydantoin usually requires

    1. sublingual therapy
    2. intramuscular therapy
    3. intravenous therapy
    4. subcutaneous therapy

386. The dose of diphenylhydantoin that may be given intravenously is

    1. 50-70 mg
    2. 50-80 mg
    3. 50-100 mg
    4. 50-120 mg

387. With which infusion rate can you avoid cardiovascular complications?

    1. 20-50 mg/min
    2. 20-40 mg/min
    3. 20-30 mg/min
    4. 10-50 mg/min

388. At what dose would you expect to see a marked hypotensive effect
from diphenylhydantoin?

    1. 100 mg
    2. 200 mg

3.   250 mg
4.   300 mg

389.   Which of the following is a reason for not administering diphenyl-
        hydantoin intramuscularly?

        1.   The procedure is too expensive.
        2.   The drug is erratically absorbed at the site.
        3.   The drug is erratically adsorbed at the site.
        4.   The drug is too unstable.

1   In open-angle glaucoma a physical blockage occurs within
        the trabecular meshwork that retards elimination of aqueous
        humor. The obstruction is presumed to be located between the
        trabecular sheet and the episcleral veins, into which the
5   aqueous humor ultimately flows. The impairment of aqueous
        drainage elevates the intraocular pressure (IOP) to 25-35 mmHg
        (normal, 10-20 mmHg), indicating that the obstruction is usu-
        ally partial. This increase in IOP is sufficient to cause
        progressive cupping of the optic disk and eventual visual
10   field defects. As the trabecular spaces become more involved,
        detachment of the cornea and formation of bullae may develop.
        In addition, scotomata (blind spots) may develop. Since vi-
        sual acuity remains largely unaffected until late in the dis-
        ease, presence of scotomata must be regarded as a major indi-
15   cation for the institution of medical therapy.

390.   Open-angle glaucoma is caused by

        1.   physical blockage
        2.   genetics
        3.   physical drainage
        4.   infection

391.   Normal IOP has a range of

        1.   10-15 mmHg
        2.   10-25 mmHg
        3.   10-20 mmHg
        4.   10-30 mmHg

392.   Increases in IOP may cause all of the following except

        1.   progressive cupping of the optic disk
        2.   visual field defects (over time)
        3.   immediate changes in visual field
        4.   development of scotomas

393.   Impairment of aqueous drainage elevates the IOP to

        1.   25-30 mmHg
        2.   25-35 mmHg
        3.   25-40 mmHg
        4.   25-45 mmHg

394. The obstruction in open-angle glaucoma is presumed to be located between

    1. the cornea and the iris
    2. the trabecular sheet and the episcleral veins
    3. the trabecular sheet and the cornea
    4. the episcleral veins and the cornea

1   An unusual reaction to quinidine is syncope. Besides
       loss of consciousness, these syncopal attacks involve pal-
       lor, muscular twitching, and sometimes seizures. When an EKG
       is obtained during an attack, the pattern indicates ventricu-
5   lar tachyarrhythmia that apparently critically decreases
       cerebral perfusion, causing loss of consciousness. The at-
       tacks usually terminate spontaneously, but the rare cases of
       sudden death attributed to quinidine are thought to be secon-
       dary to ventricular arrhythmia. On the other hand, this con-
10   dition is often observed in patients with coronary artery
       disease, where sudden death has been reported to occur as a
       result of the primary cardiac pathological condition rather
       than from the drug itself. Syncope may occur at low doses
       (e.g., 0.8 g/day) and without evidence of allergic reactions.
15   An adverse dose-related effect is hypotension, which may occur
       by alpha-adrenergic receptor blockade or by a direct negative
       inotropic effect on the heart.

395. Which of the following is not associated with syncopal attacks?

    1. pallor
    2. muscular twitching
    3. loss of consciousness
    4. itching

396. An adverse dose-related effect of quinidine is

    1. hypertension
    2. hypotension
    3. an inotropic effect
    4. diabetes

397. When an EKG is obtained during an attack, the pattern indicates

    1. arrhythmia
    2. ventricular tachyarrhythmia
    3. ventricular flutter
    4. atrial tachyarrhythmia

398. An unusual reaction to quinidine is

    1. ataxia
    2. pallor
    3. syncope
    4. hypotension

399.   Syncope may occur at

       1. high doses of quinidine
       2. moderate doses of quinidine
       3. low doses of quinidine
       4. very high doses of quinidine

1   Many reports have indicated that the tricyclic antide-
       pressants, especially imipramine, may be of benefit in the
       treatment of MBD in children. However, although most studies
       have indicated their superiority over placebos, they are
5   still not as effective as the psychostimulants. Further
       drawbacks associated with their use include the development
       of tolerance in some children and numerous deleterious side
       effects. Side effects may be somewhat limited by the maximum
       daily dose approved by the FDA (5 mg/kg per day), but the pa-
10   tient must be regularly examined for autonomic effects, weight
       loss, gastrointestinal irritation, fine tremors, hyperirrita-
       bility, and mood alterations. In addition, the patient should
       be monitored for more severe effects on the central nervous
       system, for example, seizures, and the cardiovascular system,
15   but these can usually be avoided if the practitioner adheres
       to FDA recommendations. Although the tricyclic antidepres-
       sants are helpful in the treatment of MBD in children, their
       use at this point is experimental and must be accompanied by
       certain precautions.

400.   Which of the following tricyclic antidepressants has been report-
       ed to be effective with MBD?

       1. desipramine
       2. imipramine
       3. amitriptyline
       4. doxepin

401.   The maximum daily dose approved by the FDA is

       1. 5 mg/kg per day
       2. 10 mg/kg per day
       3. 15 mg/kg per day
       4. 20 mg/kg per day

402.   While the tricyclic antidepressants are superior to placebos,
       they are still not as effective as

       1. hypnotics
       2. sedatives
       3. psychostimulants
       4. stimulants

403.   The patient must be monitored for more severe side effects on the
       central nervous system such as _____.

       1. dizziness
       2. seizures

3. headaches
4. blindness

404. Another drawback associated with the use of the tricyclics is

1. the development of addiction
2. sedation
3. the development of physical addiction
4. the development of tolerance.

1   The primary agents in the treatment of MBD are the cen-
       trally acting sympathomimetics, for example, methylphenidate,
       dextroamphetamine, and magnesium pemoline. This therapeutic
       approach was first used in 1937, but actual definition and
5   characterization of this indication in pediatric psychophar-
       macology did not become popular until the late 1960s. Dex-
       troamphetamine was initially used in 1937 and continued to be
       the agent of choice until the late 1960s, when methylphenidate
       usage increased in association with reports of a lower inci-
10   dence of side effects with the latter drug. It would appear
       that these reports of the greater safety of methylphenidate
       therapy are of questionable clinical significance. Studies
       attesting to the greater clinical efficacy of methylphenidate
       over dextroamphetamine have also been carried out by some
15   authorities who prefer the use of the former drug, while pro-
       ponents of dextroamphetamine indicate that, in their hands,
       it has comparable clinical efficacy at a lower cost.

405. The agent of choice in the treatment of MBD until the late 1960s
      was

1. amitriptyline
2. dextroamphetamine
3. methylphenidate
4. magnesium pemoline

406. Which of the following involves the lowest cost in the treatment
      of MBD?

1. dextroamphetamine
2. methylphenidate
3. amitriptyline
4. none of the above

407. Which of the following is not a primary agent in the treatment of
      MBD?

1. methylphenidate
2. magnesium pemoline
3. dextroamphetamine
4. chlorpromazine

408. Methylphenidate use increased in the late 1960s owing to reports of its

    1. lower cost
    2. decreased risk of addiction
    3. lower incidence of side effects
    4. shorter half-life

1   Procainamide may be considered as an alternative to quinidine in the treatment and prophylaxis of atrial fibrillation. Most patients absorb 75-95% of an oral dose; however, Koch-Weser estimated that 10% of subjects may absorb 50% or less.
5   This uncertainty concerning the dose absorbed and the lag time for stomach emptying into the small bowel, where the drug is finally absorbed, force the parenteral administration of procainamide in emergencies. Procainamide may be given intravenously at a rate of 25-50 mg/min. Giardina et al. have
10 intravenously administered 100 mg, up to a maximum of 1 g, every 5 min to treat ventricular arrhythmia. This method will produce a minimally effective serum concentration in 15 min. Therapy never had to be interrupted because of hypotension or conduction disturbances; however, the investigators had
15 excluded myocardial infarction patients, who are most susceptible to these adverse reactions, from their population.

409. Which of the following drugs may be considered as an alternative to quinidine?

    1. propranolol
    2. procainamide
    3. digoxin
    4. aspirin

410. The dosage used by Giardina et al. to treat ventricular arrhythmias was

    1. 100 mg intravenously every 5 min
    2. 100 mg intramuscularly every 5 min
    3. 200 mg intravenously every 5 min
    4. 200 mg intramuscularly every 5 min

411. The normal rate of intravenous administration of procainamide is

    1. 25-100 mg/min
    2. 25-75 mg/min
    3. 25-125 mg/min
    4. 25-50 mg/min

412. Most patients absorb _____ of an oral dose of procainamide.

    1. 65-75%
    2. 65-95%
    3. 75-95%
    4. 55-75%

413. Koch-Weser estimated that 10% of the patients will absorb

   1. 50% or less
   2. 60% or less
   3. 70% or less
   4. 80% or less

1   Corticosteroid-induced glaucoma is well documented. This
   form of glaucoma is usually painless and involves no ocular
   findings or visual field defects. The blockage produced prob-
   ably occurs in the trabecular meshwork, severely decreasing
5 the outflow of aqueous humor. Systemically or topically administered corticosteroids further hinder outflow, causing
   a corresponding increase in intraocular pressure. After topical therapy, a glaucomatous change occurs in the eye instilled
   with the drug. This ocular hypertensive effect is usually
10 fully reversible within 1 month after discontinuation of steroid therapy. The increase in intraocular pressure is approximately 10 mmHg for patients with preglaucomatous anterior
   chambers, and 5 mmHg for normal persons. In some cases irreversible eye damage occurs if ocular tension persists for
15 1-2 months or longer. In addition, cupping of the optic disk
   and visual field defects may develop a few months after topical administration of corticosteroids has begun. Patients
   undergoing chronic topical steroid therapy should therefore
   have a tonometric examination every 2 months.

414. The increase in intraocular pressure is approximately _____ for
   patients with preglaucomatous anterior chambers.

   1. 5 mmHg
   2. 10 mmHg
   3. 15 mmHg
   4. 20 mmHg

415. The ocular hypertensive effect caused by corticosteroids is usually

   1. irreversible
   2. fully reversible
   3. not seen
   4. partially reversible

416. Irreversible eye damage may occur if ocular hypertension persists
   for

   1. 2-4 months
   2. 1-2 months
   3. 1-4 months
   4. 2-6 months

417. Corticosteroid-induced glaucoma usually does not involve any of
   the following symptoms except

1. pain
2. physical findings in the eye
3. cupping of the optic disk
4. night blindness

418. Patients undergoing chronic topical corticosteroid therapy should have a tonometric examination every

1. month
2. 2 months
3. 3 months
4. 4 months

ANSWER KEY

Verbal Ability

1.	2		46.	1
2.	1		47.	4
3.	2		48.	2
4.	3		49.	4
5.	4		50.	4
6.	2		51.	4
7.	1		52.	2
8.	3		53.	2
9.	1		54.	2
10.	1		55.	4
11.	4		56.	4
12.	3		57.	3
13.	2		58.	4
14.	1		59.	2
15.	3		60.	3
16.	2		61.	2
17.	3		62.	1
18.	1		63.	3
19.	3		64.	4
20.	2		65.	2
21.	2		66.	2
22.	4		67.	4
23.	2		68.	1
24.	1		69.	3
25.	2		70.	2
26.	3		71.	2
27.	1		72.	4
28.	2		73.	1
29.	4		74.	4
30.	3		75.	3
31.	1		76.	2
32.	2		77.	1
33.	1		78.	3
34.	3		79	2
35.	1		80.	3
36.	3		81.	2
37.	2		82.	4
38.	3		83.	3
39.	4		84.	1
40.	1		85.	3
41.	3		86.	1
42.	4		87.	2
43.	2		88.	2
44.	2		89.	4
45.	3		90.	4

91.	2
92.	1
93.	2
94.	4
95.	3
96.	3
97.	2
98.	2
99.	4
100.	3

Quantitative Ability

101.	3		141.	1
102.	2		142.	4
103.	1		143.	2
104.	4		144.	4
105.	3		145.	4
106.	3		146.	2
107.	2		147.	3
108.	3		148.	3
109.	3		149.	1
110.	3		150.	2
111.	2		151.	1
112.	4		152.	2
113.	3		153.	2
114.	4		154.	1
115.	4		155.	4
116.	1		156.	4
117.	3		157.	1
118.	4		158.	4
119.	2		159.	2
120.	1		160.	2
121.	3		161.	3
122.	3		162.	1
123.	2		163.	3
124.	4		164.	3
125.	3		165.	3
126.	3		166.	2
127.	3		167.	2
128.	2		168.	3
129.	1		169.	3
130.	3		170.	1
131.	3		171.	4
132.	2		172.	4
133.	3		173.	1
134.	1		174.	3
135.	4		175.	1
136.	2		176.	2
137.	1		177.	2
138.	1		178.	4
139.	4		179.	1
140.	2		180.	3

181.	3		191.	4
182.	4		192.	1
183.	1		193.	2
184.	2		194.	4
185.	3		195.	4
186.	4		196.	1
187.	1		197.	2
188.	1		198.	4
189.	1		199.	3
190.	2		200.	1

Biology

201.	3		243.	3
202.	2		244.	2
203.	2		245.	3
204.	3		246.	2
205.	4		247.	1
206.	4		248.	3
207.	2		249.	4
208.	1		250.	1
209.	1		251.	4
210.	3		252.	3
211.	4		253.	3
212.	2		254.	1
213.	1		255.	4
214.	3		256.	1
215.	2		257.	2
216.	1		258.	3
217.	2		259.	4
218.	3		260.	1
219.	4		261.	3
220.	2		262.	1
221.	4		263.	4
222.	1		264.	2
223.	4		265.	3
224.	3		266.	4
225.	2		267.	3
226.	3		268.	1
227.	3		269.	2
228.	4		270.	4
229.	1		271.	3
230.	3		272.	4
231.	1		273.	1
232.	4		274.	3
233.	2		275.	1
234.	2			
235.	3			
236.	4			
237.	3			
238.	1			
239.	4			
240.	4			
241.	1			
242.	3			

Chemistry

276.	4	326.	1
277.	2	327.	3
278.	4	328.	2
279.	1	329.	1
280.	2	330.	1
281.	2	331.	1
282.	2	332.	2
283.	1	333.	2
284.	3	334.	2
285.	2	335.	2
286.	2	336.	4
287.	3	337.	1
288.	3	338.	2
289.	3	339.	3
290.	4	340.	4
291.	4	341.	1
292.	1	342.	2
293.	4	343.	3
294.	1	344.	4
295.	4	345.	4
296.	3	346.	3
297.	1	347.	2
298.	4	348.	1
299.	4	349.	3
300.	1	350.	1
301.	1	351.	2
302.	1	352.	4
303.	2	353.	4
304.	4	354.	3
305.	3	355.	2
306.	3	356.	4
307.	4	357.	3
308.	2	358.	2
309.	1	359.	1
310.	3	360.	2
311.	3	361.	3
312.	3	362.	4
313.	4	363.	4
314.	1	364.	1
315.	4	365.	3
316.	3	366.	2
317.	4	367.	4
318.	2	368.	3
319.	3	369.	3
320.	3	370.	1
321.	1	371.	2
322.	4	372.	3
323.	1	373.	4
324.	4	374.	2
325.	1	375.	1

Reading Comprehension

376.	4		401.	1
377.	2		402.	3
378.	1		403.	2
379.	2		404.	4
380.	2		405.	2
381.	3		406.	1
382.	2		407.	4
383.	3		408.	3
384.	4		409.	2
385.	3		410.	1
386.	3		411.	4
387.	1		412.	3
388.	4		413.	1
389.	2		414.	2
390.	1		415.	2
391.	3		416.	2
392.	3		417.	3
393.	2		418.	2
394.	2			
395.	4			
396.	2			
397.	2			
398.	3			
399.	3			
400.	2			

EXPLANATORY ANSWERS

Verbal Ability

The verbal ability answers include the basic definition of the word and the corresponding correct answer (the word that means either the same or most nearly the same for Questions 1-50, and the word which is opposite in meaning for Questions 51-100), as well as whether it is a noun (n), pronoun (p), verb (v), or adjective (a).

1. EXTENT (n)--the range over which something extends.
Ans. (2) width (n)--largeness of extent or scope.

2. AWAKE (v)--roused from or as if from sleep.
Ans. (1) arouse (v)--to awaken from sleep.

3. TACT (n)--a keen sense of what to do or say in order to maintain good relations with others.
Ans. (2) diplomacy (n)--the art and practice of conducting negotiations or affairs without arousing hostility.

4. EXPERT (n)--one who has acquired special skill in or knowledge and mastery of something.
Ans. (3) authority (n)--an individual recognized for his or her knowledge in a particular area.

5. ACCOUNT (n)--chronological record of debit and credit entries posted to a ledger page; a statement of transactions during a fiscal period.
Ans. (4) statement (n)--a summary of a financial account showing the balance due.

6. ACCRUE (v)--to periodically accumulate, whether as an increase or a decrease.
Ans. (2) accumulate (v)--to heap or pile up; to increase in number.

7. BULLETIN (n)--a brief public notice issuing from an authoritive source.
Ans. (1) announcement (n)--a public notification or declaration.

8. BRIDLE (n)--something that restrains in the same fashion as the headgear with which a horse is governed.
Ans. (3) control (n)--an act or instance of controlling; the power or authority to guide or manage.

9. CONTAMINATE (v)--to debase by making impure or unclean.
Ans. (1) pollute (v)--to make physically impure or unclean.

10. DISPLEASURE (n)--the feeling of one who is displeased.
Ans. (1) pique (n)--a transient feeling of wounded vanity; a fit of resentment.

11. EVENTUATE (v)--to come out finally; to result.
Ans. (4) ensue (v)--to take place afterward or as a result.

12. MAGNIFICENCE (n)--the quality
    or state of being magnifi-
    cent; the splendor of sur-
    roundings.
    Ans. (3) grandiosity (n)--
    --splendor; affectation of
    grandeur.

13. UNDULATE (v)--to form or move
    in waves.
    Ans. (2) slither (v)--to
    slide on or as if on a
    loose, gravelly surface;
    to slip or slide like a
    snake.

14. PARSIMONIOUS (a)--frugal to
    the point of stinginess.
    Ans. (1) niggardly (a)--ex-
    cessively mean about spend-
    ing or giving.

15. QUIESCENT (a)--becoming quiet;
    at rest; inactive.
    Ans. (3) immobile (a)--in-
    capable of being moved; not
    moving.

16. RADIOACTIVITY (n)--the prop-
    erty possessed by some el-
    ements (such as uranium)
    of spontaneously emitting
    alpha, beta, and/or gamma
    rays by the disintegration
    of atomic nuclei.
    Ans. (2) radiation (n)--the
    process of emitting radi-
    ant energy in the form of
    waves or particles.

17. COLLEGIAN (n)--a student or
    recent college graduate.
    Ans. (3) student (n)--an in-
    dividual who attends school.

18. FLANK (n)--the right or left
    side of a formation; a cut
    of meat.
    Ans. (1) side (n)--the right
    or left part of the wall or
    trunk of the body.

19. DIPSOMANIAC (n)--an individ-
    ual with an uncontrollable
    craving for alcoholic bev-
    erages.

Ans. (3) alcoholic (n)--one
affected with alcoholism.

20. CORSAGE (n)--an arrangement
    of flowers to be worn by a
    woman.
    Ans. (2) nosegay (n)--a small
    bunch of flowers.

21. CORTEGE (n)--a train of at-
    tendants.
    Ans. (2) retinue (n)--a group
    of retainers or attendants.

22. JOWL (n)--jaw; one of the
    lateral halves of the man-
    dible; cheek.
    Ans. (4) jaw (n)--either of two
    bony structures in most
    vertebrates that border the
    mouth.

23. SUPREMACY (n)--the quality or
    state of being supreme; su-
    preme authority or power.
    Ans. (2) chieftaincy (n)--
    the rank, dignity, office,
    or role of a chieftain.

24. PLIABLE (a)--supple enough to
    bend freely or repeatedly
    without breaking;
    rapidly to others.
    Ans. (1) flexible (a)--capa-
    ble of being flexed; pliant.

25. ZEALOT (n)--a member of a
    fanatical sect arising in
    Judea; a zealous person; a
    fanatical partisan.
    Ans. (2) fanatic (n)--a fol-
    lower of a cause who is
    characterized by excessive
    enthusiasm and often intense
    uncritical devotion.

26. TRANSCEND (v)--to rise above
    or go beyond the limits of.
    Ans. (3) exceed (v)--to ex-
    tend outside of; to be
    greater than or superior to;
    to go beyond a limit.

27. SHREWD (a)--marked by clever,
    discerning awareness and
    hard-headed acumen; given

to wily and artful ways of
dealing.
Ans. (1) cagey (a)--hesitant
about committing oneself;
wary of being trapped or
deceived; shrewd.

28. EXPENDITURE (n)--the act or
process of expending; something expended; disburse-
ment; expense.
Ans. (2) disbursement (n)--
the act of disbursing.

29. EXPEDIENCY (n)--the quality
or state of being suited
to the end in view.
Ans. (4) appropriateness (n)--
especially suitable or
compatible; fitting.

30. SILKEN (a)--made or consist-
ing of silk; agreeably
smooth; extremely elegant.
Ans. (3) luxurious (a)--of
or relating to unrestrained
gratification of the senses;
of the finest and richest
kind.

31. DEPART (v)--to go away; to
turn aside; to swerve.
Ans. (1) withdraw (v)--to
take back or away.

32. DENOUNCE (v)--to pronounce,
especially publically,
someone to be blameworthy
or evil; to inform against.
Ans. (2) impeach (v)--to
bring an accusation against;
to charge with a crime or
misdemeanor.

33. DENUDE (v)--to strip of all
covering; to lay bare by
erosion.
Ans. (1) peel (v)--to remove
by stripping.

34. FLYSPECK (n)--a speck made
by fly excrement; something
small and insignificant.
Ans. (3) speckle (n)-- a little speck; a very small
amount.

35. DEVIATORY (a)--straying, especially from a standard, principle, or topic.
Ans. (1) aberrant (a)--stray-
ing from the correct or normal way; deviating from the
usual or natural kind.

36. MELEE (n)--a confused struggle;
a hand-to-hand fight among
several people.
Ans. (3) skirmish (n)--a minor
fight in war, usually inci-
dental to a larger movement;
a minor dispute or contest
between opposing parties.

37. MEDICAMENT (n)--a substance
used in therapy.
Ans. (2) medicine (n)--a substance used in treating
disease.

38. PALPABLE (a)--capable of
being touched or felt;
tangible; easily percepti-
ble.
Ans. (3)touchable (a)--able to
be touched or handled.

39. RUDIMENTARY (a)--consisting
in first principles; of a
primitive kind.
Ans. (4) basal (a)--relating
to the situation at or forming the base.

40. TONICITY (n)--the property
of possessing tone, especially healthy vigor of body
and mind.
Ans. (1) tone (n)--healthy
elasticity.

41. VALIDATE (v)--make legally
valid; to grant official
sanction to by marking.
Ans. (3) authenticate (v)--
to prove or serve to prove
the authenticity of.

42. TARIFF (n)--a schedule of du-
ties imposed on imported or
exported goods.
Ans. (4) duty (n)--a tax on
imports.

43. WARBLE (n)--a melodious succession of low pleasing sounds; a musical trill.
Ans. (2) diapason (n)--a burst of harmonious sound.

44. YAHOO (n)--a member of a race of brutes in Swift's Gulliver's Travels who have the form and all the vices of man; an uncouth or rowdy person.
Ans. (2) ruffian (n)--a brutal person; a bully.

45. SUAVE (a)--smoothly though often superficially affable and polite; smooth in performance or finish.
Ans. (3) urbane (a)--notably polite or finished in manner; polished; suave.

46. REMORSELESS (a)--having no remorse; merciless; persistent and indefatigable.
Ans. (1) impenitent (a)--not penitent.

47. PERSNICKETY (a)--fussy about small details; having the characteristics of a snob.
Ans. (4) fastidious (a)--having high and often capricious standards; showing or demanding excessive delicacy or care.

48. PERIMETER (n)--the boundary of a closed plane figure; outer limits.
Ans. (2) periphery (n)--the external boundary of a body; the perimeter of something.

49. IMPERIOUS (a)--befitting or characteristic of eminent rank or attainments; marked by arrogant assurance; compelling.
Ans. (4) domineering--masterful; characterized by overbearing control.

50. COMPASSION (n)--sympathetic understanding of others'
distress together with a desire to alleviate it.
Ans. (4) clemency (n)--the disposition to be merciful and especially to moderate the severity of punishment due.

51. DIFFICULTY (n)--the quality or state of being difficult; something difficult.
Ans. (4) effortlessness (n)--showing or requiring little or no effort.

52. IDEALISM (n)--the theory that true reality lies in a realm beyond phenomena; the practice of forming ideals or living under their influence.
Ans. (2) realism (n)--concern for fact or reality and rejection of the impractical and visionary.

53. HYSTERICAL (a)--characterized by unmanageable fear or emotional excess.
Ans. (2) calm (a)--still; free from agitation, excitement, or disturbance.

54. WELCOME (n)--a greeting or cordial remark made upon the entrance or arrival of a guest.
Ans. (2) goodbye (n)--an ending remark made to one who is leaving.

55. SILVER (n)--one of the elements that is a metal.
Ans. (4) xenon--one of the elements that is a gas.

56. EXTRANEOUS (a)--existing on the outside; not forming an essential part.
Ans. (4) intrinsic (a)--belonging to the essential nature of a thing.

57. FACTORY (n)--a place where goods are manufactured.
Ans. (3) store (n)-- a place where goods can be purchased.

58. TAME (a)--calm or changed from a state of being wild to a domestic state.
Ans. (4) fierce (a)--wild and hostile in temperament; given to fighting.

59. MAELSTROM (n)--a powerful, often violent whirlpool sucking in objects within a given radius.
Ans. (2) steadiness (n)-- showing little variation or fluctuation.

60. NEFARIOUS (a)--flagrantly wicked or impious.
Ans. (3) generous (a)--characterized by a noble or forbearing spirit.

61. OPINION (n)--a judgment formed in the mind about a particular matter.
Ans. (2) operation (n)--performance of something involving the practical application of principles.

62. PARALLEL (a)--extending everywhere in the same direction and not meeting.
Ans. (1) vertical (a)--perpendicular to a primary axis.

63. QUASH (v)--to nullify, to suppress summarily and completely.
Ans. (3) initiate (v)--to cause the beginning of; to introduce.

64. QUAY (n)--a solid, man-made landing place constructed by navigable water for ease in loading and unloading ships.
Ans. (4) harbor (n)--a part of a protected body of water that is deep enough to furnish anchorage.

65. ANIMATION (n)--the act of giving life or spirit to.
Ans. (2) evisceration (n)--the taking away of vital force.

66. REMONSTRATION (n)--protestation; presentation of reasons for opposition.
Ans. (2) acquiescence (n)--the act of accepting without objection.

67. ECLECTIC (a)--composed of elements drawn from various sources.
Ans. (4) homogeneous (a)--of uniform structure throughout.

68. FAMOUS (a)--honored for outstanding achievement; widely known.
Ans. (1) undistinguished (a)--not marked by any distinction.

69. GLUTTONOUS (a)--excessive in eating or drinking.
Ans. (3) abstemious (a)--sparing, especially in eating or drinking.

70. GLOAMING (n)--twilight.
Ans. (2) morning (n)--dawn; the time from sunrise to noon.

71. GNOME (n)--a folkloric creature.
Ans. (2) human (n)--a human being.

72. GLIMPSE (v)--to take a brief look.
Ans. (4) peer (v)--to look searchingly at something to discern.

73. GLOOMY (a)--partially or totally dark; dismally dark.
Ans. (1) gloomless (a)--without gloom.

74. INTONATION (n)--the act of uttering something either in single tones or in monotone.
Ans. (4) inarticulateness (n)--the inability to express something by speech.

75. JOVIALITY (n)--state of being markedly good humored, convivial, merry.
Ans. (3) melancholy (n)--depression.

76. SAGE (n)--one distinguished for wisdom and sound judgment.
Ans. (2) temerariousness (n)--temerity; rash or presumptious daring.

77. LISSOME (a)--lithe or nimble.
Ans. (1) rigid (a)--not flexible; stiff and unyielding.

78. OBDURATE (a)--hardened in feelings; resistant to persuasion or softening influences.
Ans. (3) tender (a)--having a soft or yielding nature.

79. OBSTREPEROUS (a)--unruly; marked by unruliness or aggressiveness.
Ans. (2) whist (a)--quiet, silent.

80. VALEDICTION (n)--a goodbye; the act of saying farewell.
Ans. (3) greeting (n)--a reception or welcome.

81. OPEN-AIR (a)--outdoor.
Ans. (2) inside (a)--of, relating to, or being on or near the inside.

82. HUMANOID (a)--having human form or character.
Ans. (4) animal-like (a)--like an animal, as distinguished from man.

83. BUOYANCY (n)--the tendency of a body to float or rise when submerged in a fluid; the ability to quickly recover from depression.
Ans. (3) sinkage (n)--the process or degree of sinking.

84. BURGH (n)--an ancient walled city; a city.
Ans. (1) camp (n)--temporary shelter.

85. ENTHRALLED (a)--to be held spellbound or to be captivated by something.
Ans. (3) free (a)--not constrained or dominated by another; independent.

86. SENILE (a)--exhibiting a loss of mental faculties associated with old age.
Ans. (1) keen (a)--showing quick and ardent responsiveness.

87. TELESTHETIC (a)--an impression received at a distance, supposedly without the normal operation of the sense organs.
Ans. (2) telephonic (a)--conveyed by telephone.

88. TEMERITY (n)--unreasonable or foolhardy contempt of danger or opposition; rashness; recklessness.
Ans. (2) caution (n)--warning; admonishment; prudent forethought to minimize risk.

89. POLYCHROMATIC (a)--displaying a variety or a change of colors; multicolored.
Ans. (4) monochromatic (a)--of one color.

90. MODIFY (v)--to make changes in.
Ans. (4) continue (v)--to keep the same; to maintain without interruption.

91. FURORE (n)--an outburst of public indignation.
Ans. (2) applause (n)--publicly expressed approval.

92. CONCILIATE (v)--to make compatible; reconcile.
Ans. (1) antagonize (v)--to incur or provoke the hostility of.

93. DESCENDANT (n)--one descended
    from another.
    Ans. (2) ancestor (n)--a per-
    son from whom one is de-
    scended.

94. FAIR (n)--free from bias;
    equitable.
    Ans. (4) biased (a)--prej-
    udiced.

95. LASCIVIOUS (a)--lewd, lustful.
    Ans. (3) puritan (a)--rela-
    ting to the Puritans or
    puritanism; morally strict.

96. PURCHASABLE (a)--available;
    within the ability to pur-
    chase or buy.
    Ans. (3) unavailable (a)--
    not available.

97. RESTITUTE (v)--to restore to
    a former state or position;
    to give back.
    Ans. (2) take (v)--to get
    into one's hands or into
    one's possession, power,
    or control.

98. MEDLEY (a)--mixed or motley.
    Ans. (2) uniform (a)--not
    varying; similar in appear-
    ance, pattern, or color.

99. IMPROMPTU (a)--on the spur
    of the moment; improvised;
    extemporaneous.
    Ans. (4) rehearsed (a)--
    practiced beforehand.

100. WHIMSICAL (a)--capricious;
     impulsive.
     Ans. (3) steadfast--immova-
     ble; not subject to change.

Quantitative Ability

101. Ans. (3)

To add or subtract fractions to equivalent fractions with the same least common denominator (LCD):

$$\frac{3}{8} + \frac{4}{5} = \frac{3 \times 5}{8 \times 5} + \frac{4 \times 8}{5 \times 8}$$

$$= \frac{15}{40} + \frac{32}{40}$$

$$= \frac{47}{40}$$

$$= 1\frac{7}{40}$$

102. Ans. (2)

To add or subtract arithmetic fractions and decimal fractions, convert to a common base:

$$0.25 + \frac{15}{16} = \frac{4}{16} + \frac{15}{16}$$

$$= \frac{19}{16}$$

$$= 1\frac{3}{16}$$

or

$$0.25 + \frac{15}{16} = 0.25 + 0.9375$$

$$= 1.1875$$

103. Ans. (1)

The following relations may be used when dealing with scientific notation:

$$10^0 = 1$$
$$10^{-A} = \frac{1}{10^A}$$
$$10^{A+B} = 10^A \times 10^B$$
$$\frac{10^A}{10^B} = 10^{A-B}$$
$$(10^A)^B = 10^{AB}$$

Therefore since

$1.30 = 1.30 \times 10^0$

and

$236 = 2.36 \times 10^2$

we have

$(1.30 \times 10^0) \times (2.36 \times 10^2) = 3.068 \times 10^{0+2}$

$$= 3.068 \times 10^2$$

104. <u>Ans. (4)</u>

The log of a product equals the sum of the logs of the component numbers:

$\log (50 \times 2) = \log 50 + \log 2 = \log 2 + \log 50$

105. <u>Ans. (3)</u>

The logs of multiples of 10, for example, 1, 10, 0.1, are integers:

10^2	$= 100,$	$\log 100$	$= 2$
10^1	$= 10,$	$\log 10$	$= 1$
10^0	$= 1,$	$\log 1$	$= 0$
10^{-1}	$= 0.1,$	$\log 0.01$	$= -1$
10^{-2}	$= 0.01$	$\log 0.01$	$= -2$
10^{-3}	$= 0.001$	$\log 0.001$	$= -3$

106. <u>Ans. (3)</u>

The root of a power is found by dividing the exponent of the power by the index of the root (see the law of exponents in Answer 119):

$8^{1/3}$ 8 is the power

1 is the exponent

3 is the root

$= \sqrt[3]{8}$

107. <u>Ans. (2)</u>

The log of a number is the exponent of the power to which a given base must be raised in order to equal that number; that is, if

$Y = a^X$

then

$\log_a Y = X$

Therefore

$\log_{10} 1000 = 3$

or base 10 raised to the third power equals 1000.

108. Ans. (3)

When adding or subtracting in scientific notation, convert to the same exponent, then add the products; the exponent will remain constant:

$1 \times 10^{-2} = 0.01 \times 10^{0}$

and

$2.3 \times 10^{1} = 23 \times 10^{0}$

So

$(0.01 \times 10^{0}) + (23 \times 10^{0}) = 23.01 \times 10^{0}$

$$= 23.01$$

109. Ans. (3)

Percent, written as %, means per hundred. It is a type of ratio and thus has no units. To express a fraction as a percentage, set 100 as the denominator and multiply by 100%:

$\frac{3}{16} \times 100\% = 0.1875 \times 100\%$

$$= 18.75\%$$

110. Ans. (3)

Weight-per-volume measurements are often expressed as percentages. To calculate the percent weight per volume, convert the fraction to a percentage, that is, with a denominator of 100, times 100%:

$\frac{2.3 \text{ g}}{10 \text{ ml}} = \frac{23 \text{ g}}{100 \text{ ml}}$

and

$\frac{23 \text{ g}}{100 \text{ ml}} \times 100\% = 23\% \text{ wt/vol}$

111.   Ans. (2)

This problem involves the use of two ratios set equal to one another to form an equation known as a proportion. To solve a proportion only one number may be unknown, which will be called $\underline{X}$. To solve, rearrange the equation such that $\underline{X}$ remains alone. Given A:B = C:D, the following rules may be used:

1.   The product of the means equals the product of the extremes: $\underline{B}$ x $\underline{C}$ = $\underline{A}$ x $\underline{D}$.

2.   The product of the means divided by one extreme gives the other extreme: $\dfrac{BC}{A}$ = $\underline{D}$.

3.   The product of the extremes divided by one mean gives the other mean: $\dfrac{AD}{B}$ = $\underline{C}$.

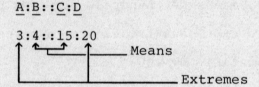

Therefore

4% solution = $\dfrac{4\ g}{100\ ml}$ from Answer 110

and

$\underline{X}$ = number of liters in which 24 g will be dissolved.

(Note: 1000 ml = 1 liter.) Since

4 g:100 ml::24 g:$\underline{X}$ ml

then

$$\frac{4\ g}{100\ ml} = \frac{24\ g}{\underline{X}}$$

$$\underline{X} = \frac{24\ g\ x\ 100\ ml}{4\ g}$$

= 600 ml

= 0.6 liter

112.   Ans. (4)

This problem is similar to that of Question 111 in that a proportionality is needed to solve the problem. First determine the total number of grams of NaCl that will be used to make the 0.9% solution:

$$18\% = \frac{18 \text{ g}}{100 \text{ ml}} \text{ x } 1000 \text{ ml}$$

$$= 180 \text{ g}$$

This quantity will be diluted with the final total volume, the unknown X, which should result in a 0.9% solution:

$$0.9\% = \frac{0.9 \text{ g}}{100 \text{ ml}}$$

and

$$\frac{0.9 \text{ g}}{100 \text{ ml}} = \frac{180 \text{ g}}{X \text{ ml}}$$

so

$$X \text{ ml} = \frac{180 \text{ g x } 100 \text{ ml}}{0.9 \text{ g}}$$

$$= 20,000 \text{ ml}$$

$$= 20 \text{ liters}$$

113.   Ans. (3)

When one mixes different strengths, the units and types of percent (wt/wt, wt/vol, vol/vol) must be kept constant. Determine the total amount of alcohol in all solutions and the total amount of solution, assuming additivity of volumes on mixing. Then convert to the desired final ratio:

25% x 5000 ml = 1250 ml

50% x 2000 ml = 1000 ml

$$10\% \text{ x } \frac{50 \text{ ml}}{7500 \text{ ml}} = \frac{50 \text{ ml}}{2300 \text{ ml}} \text{ ethanol}$$

So

$$\frac{2300 \text{ ml of ethanol}}{7500 \text{ ml of solution}} = 0.3067 \cong 30.7\%$$

114. <u>Ans. (4)</u>

The laws of logarithms are derived from the laws of exponents (see Answer 119). The most commonly used base is 10, although any base may be used.

$\log(\underline{ab}) = \log \underline{a} + \log \underline{b}$

$\log(\underline{a}/\underline{b}) = \log \underline{a} - \log \underline{b}$

$\log \underline{a}^{\underline{n}} = \underline{n} \times \log \underline{a}$

$\log \underline{a}^{1/\underline{n}} = \log \sqrt[\underline{n}]{\underline{a}} = (1/\underline{n}) \log \underline{a}$

Therefore

$\log \sqrt{25} = 1/2 \log 25 = \dfrac{(\log 25)}{2}$

$\qquad\qquad = \log 25^{\frac{1}{2}}$

$\qquad\qquad = \log 5$

115. <u>Ans. (4)</u>

From previous answers,

$\log \underline{a}^{\underline{n}} = \underline{n} \times \log \underline{a}$

$\log 25^{2} = 2 \times \log 25$

116. <u>Ans. (1)</u>

This problem involves ratios. First convert to common units:

1 kg = 1000 g

Then set up the proportionality:

$$\frac{1 \text{ kg}}{2.2 \text{ lb}} = \frac{X}{1 \text{ lb}}$$

$$\frac{1000 \text{ g} \times (1 \text{ lb})}{2.2 \text{ lb}} = X$$

454.5 g = X

117. <u>Ans. (3)</u>

Whenever mathematical procedures are used, all the units must be the

same. Therefore

1 liter = 1000 ml

and

1000 ml - 283 ml = 717 ml

118. <u>Ans. (4)</u>

See Answers 111 and 116.

Since

1 g   = 1000 mg

we have

$$\frac{15.43 \text{ grains}}{1000 \text{ mg}} = \frac{1 \text{ grain}}{X \text{ mg}}$$

$$\underline{X} \text{ mg} = \frac{1 \text{ grain} \times 1000 \text{ mg}}{15.43 \text{ grains}}$$

$\underline{X}$ = 64.81 mg

119. <u>Ans. (2)</u>

First simplify the numbers (see Answer 106); then use the law of ex-

ponents:

1. The product of two or more powers of the <u>same base</u> is the base
    with an exponent equal to the <u>sum of all the exponents</u>:
    $$4^3 \times 4^{10} = 4^{10+3} = 4^{13}$$

2. The quotient of two powers with the <u>same base</u> is the base
    with an exponent equal to the <u>exponent of the numerator</u>
    <u>minus that of the denominator</u>:
    $$\frac{3^8}{3^2} = 3^{8-2} = 3^6$$

3. The power of a power is found by <u>multiplying the exponents</u>:
    $$(2^4)^3 = 2^{4 \times 3} = 2^{12}$$

4. The power of a product equals the <u>product of the powers</u> of the factors:

$$(2 \times 3 \times 4)^2 = 2^2 \times 3^2 \times 4^2$$

5. The root of a power is found by <u>dividing the exponent of the power by the index of the root</u>:

$$\sqrt[3]{8^6} = 8^{6/3} = 8^2$$

6. The power of a fraction equals the <u>power of the numerator divided by the power of the denominator</u>:

$$(2/3)^2 = \frac{2^2}{3^2}$$

7. A number with a <u>negative</u> exponent equals 1 divided by the number with a positive exponent:

$$12^{-2} = \frac{1}{12^2}$$

8. Any number other than 0 with exponent 0 equals 1:

$$10^0 = 1, \qquad 4^0 = 1, \qquad 1^0 = 1$$

Therefore for Problem 119 we have

$$\sqrt[3]{3^6} = 3^{6/3} = 3^2$$

and

$$\sqrt{2^2} = 2^{2/2} = 2^1 = 2$$

so

$$3^2 + 2 = (3 \times 3) + 2$$

$$3^2 + 2 = 11$$

120. <u>Ans. (1)</u>

From above, making the appropriate conversion to the least common denominator, we have

$$(2/3)^2 + 2^{-3} = \frac{2^2}{3^2} + \frac{1}{2^3}$$

$$= 4/9 + 1/8$$

$$= \frac{4 \times 8}{9 \times 8} + \frac{9 \times 1}{9 \times 8}$$

$$= 32/72 + 9/72$$

$$= 41/72$$

121. <u>Ans. (3)</u>

From above, we have

$10° = 1$

$10^1 = 10$

$10^{-1} = 0.1$
_____

11.1

122. <u>Ans. (3)</u>

In problems involving formulas, rearrange the formula until the unknown
term is expressed by all the other terms. Therefore if the temperature
in degrees centigrade is unknown, rearrange the formula as follows:

$9(\underline{X}°C) = 5(\underline{Y}°F) - 160$

$\underline{X}°C \quad = 5/9(\underline{Y}°F) - 160/9$

$$= \frac{5 \times 79}{9} - 17.78$$

$$= 26.1$$

123. <u>Ans. (2)</u>

Rearrange to solve for the temperature in degrees Fahrenheit as
explained above:

$9(\underline{X}°C) = 5(\underline{Y}°F) - 160$

$5(\underline{Y}°F) = 9(\underline{X}°C) + 160$

$\underline{Y}°F \quad = 9/5(\underline{X}°C) + 160/5$

$$= \frac{9 \times (-10)}{5} + 32$$

$$= -18 + 32$$

$$= 14$$

124. Ans. (4)

This problem may be approached by determining the respective temperatures in degrees centigrade and then computing the difference. From

$$X°C = \frac{5(Y°F) - 160}{9}$$

we have

$$X°C = \frac{5(72) - 160}{9}, \quad X'°C = \frac{5(65) - 160}{9}$$

$$X°C = 22.22, \quad X'°C \cong 18.33$$

So

$$22.22 - 18.33 \cong 3.88 \quad 3.9°C$$

Alternately, as one degree Fahrenheit is 9/5 of a degree on the centigrade scale, the problem may be solved by multiplying the differences in degrees Farenheit by 5/9.

$$72°F - 65°F = 7°F$$

$$7°F \times \frac{5}{9} = \frac{35}{9} = 3.88°C$$

You cannot directly substitute the 7°F into the temperature conversion equation as originally given, since that equation converts the 7°F to the corresponding temperature in degrees centigrade. That is, 7°F equals -13.8°C.

125. Ans. (3)

This is a proportionality problem. Assume a weight-volume relationship 1:10,000::X:200:

$$\frac{1 \text{ g}}{10,000 \text{ ml}} = \frac{X \text{ g}}{200 \text{ ml}}$$

$$X \text{ g} = \frac{(1 \text{ g}) \times (200 \text{ ml})}{10,000 \text{ ml}}$$

$$= 0.02 \text{ g}$$

126. **Ans. (3)**

When $\underline{X}$ is known, $\underline{Y}$ may be found by drawing a line up from the $\underline{X}$ axis, parallel to the $\underline{Y}$ axis, until the line of the graph is intersected. A line is then drawn from this point perpendicular to the $\underline{Y}$ axis until it is intersected. This is the value of $\underline{Y}$ for a given $\underline{X}$.

127. **Ans. (3)**

The rate of drug disappearance is the change in $\underline{Y}$ (mg drug/ml plasma) over a range of $\underline{X}$ (time). This is equal to the slope

$$\frac{\underline{Y}_2 - \underline{Y}_1}{\underline{X}_2 - \underline{X}_1} = \underline{m}$$

Therefore, to determine the rate (slope), any two $\underline{Y}$ values and corresponding $\underline{X}$ values are needed: For example,

$$\text{time}_1 = 0 \text{ min}, \qquad Y_1 = \frac{\text{mg drug}}{\text{ml plasma}} = 4$$

$$\text{time}_2 = 80 \text{ min}, \qquad Y_2 = \frac{\text{mg drug}}{\text{ml plasma}} = 2$$

Then

$$\text{rate} = \frac{2-4}{80-0} = \frac{-2}{80} = \frac{-1}{40}$$

and

$$\frac{-1}{40} = \frac{-1 \text{ mg/ml plasma}}{40 \text{ min}} = -1.5 \text{ mg/ml plasma per hour}$$

Note: The negative sign indicates a decline, or falling $\underline{Y}$ values, for increasing $\underline{X}$ values.

128. **Ans. (2)**

To predict a $\underline{Y}$ value for a given $\underline{X}$, the slope $\underline{m}$ and the $\underline{Y}$ intercept $\underline{b}$ must be known so we can solve $\underline{Y} = \underline{m}\underline{X} + \underline{b}$. From Answer 128,

$$\underline{m} = \frac{-1.5 \text{ mg/ml plasma}}{1 \text{ hr.}}$$

and

b = 4 mg/ml plasma

$\underline{X}$ = 2 hr

So

$\underline{Y}$ = (-1.5 mg/ml per hour x (2 hr) + 4 mg/ml

  = -3.0 mg/ml + 4 mg/ml

  = 1.0 mg/ml

Remember to include the negative sign in the slope.

129. Ans. (1)

In this problem the $\underline{Y}$ intercept has been changed to 8 mg/ml and the time to 80 min (1.33 hr). The problem is then solved as above:

$\underline{Y}$ = $\underline{mX}$ + $\underline{b}$

  = (-1.5 mg/ml per hour x (1.33 hr) + 8 mg/hr

  = -1.995 + 8

$\cong$ 6 mg/ml

130. Ans. (3)

This problem requires finding the value of $\underline{X}$ (time) when $\underline{Y}$ (concentration) is zero. Again,

$\underline{Y}$ is $\underline{mX}$ + $\underline{b}$

0 = (-1.5 mg/ml per hour)$\underline{X}$ + 4 mg/ml

$\dfrac{-\ 4\ mg/ml}{-1.5\ mg/ml\ per\ hour}$ = $\underline{X}$

2.66 hr   = $\underline{X}$

160 min   = $\underline{X}$

131. Ans. (3)

An integer is any of the natural numbers, the negatives of the numbers and zero. To find the values for the inequalities, solve each of the inequalities separately; then delete all values not satisfying both:

$4 < 3\underline{x}-2 \leq 10$	$3\underline{x} - 2 \leq 10$
$4 < 3\underline{x}-2$	$3\underline{x} \leq 10 + 2$
$4 + 2\ 3\underline{x}$	$3\underline{x} \leq 12$
$6/3 < \underline{x}$	$\underline{x} \leq 4$
$2 < \underline{x}$	

Therefore all values greater than 2 may be accepted: 3, 4, 5, ..., $\underline{n}$	Therefore all values less than or equal to 4 will be accepted: 4, 3, 2, 1, 0, -1, -2, ..., -$\underline{n}$

Integer values common to both inequalities are 3 and 4.

132. <u>Ans. (2)</u>

$\dfrac{7}{\underline{x}} > 2, \quad \underline{x} \neq 0$

$7 > 2\underline{x}$

$7/2 > x$

$3.5 > \underline{x}$

$\underline{x}$ must be less than 3.5, or 3, 2, 1, 0, -1, -2, ..., but $\underline{x}$ cannot be 0; therefore 3, 2, 1 are common to both equations.

133. <u>Ans. (3)</u>

The absolute value $|\underline{X}|$ removes the sign of the number enclosed after all arithmetic functions enclosed have been completed, or $|-\underline{X}| = \underline{X}$. Therefore

$|-5| - |-2| = 5 - 2 = 3$

134. <u>Ans. (1)</u>

$|8 - 14| = |-6| = 6$

135. Ans. (4)

$|5\underline{x} + 4| = -3$

This problem cannot be solved, as there is no term whose absolute value will yield a negative result.

136. <u>Ans. (2)</u>

As the figure is a cube, <u>D</u> is the hypotenuse of a right triangle with equal sides. From the Pythagorean theorem, we have

hypotenuse^2 = side^2 + side'^{2}

$$\underline{x}^2 = 2^2 + 2^2$$
$$\underline{x}^2 = 4 + 4$$
$$\underline{x}^2 = 8$$
$$X = \sqrt{8}$$

137. <u>Ans. (1)</u>

In this example, lines <u>C</u>, <u>D</u>, and <u>E</u> form a right triangle with base <u>D</u> and side <u>C</u> (or base <u>C</u> and side <u>D</u>). If <u>C</u> is 2 in. (given condition) and <u>D</u> from the previous example is $\sqrt{8}$ in., then $1/2 \sqrt{8}(2) = \sqrt{8}$ in.^{2} (The area of a triangle is equal to 1/2 base x height.) <u>E</u> could also serve as a base, except, as <u>E</u> was unknown, it was easier to work with the sides already known.

138. <u>Ans. (1)</u>

A cube has six faces: top, bottom, and four sides. If each face has a surface area of 2 x 2 in.^{2}, then the total area is

$\frac{(2 \text{ in. x 2 in.})}{\text{face}}$ x 6 faces = 24 in.^{2}

139. <u>Ans. (4)</u>

The subset of "<u>A</u> or <u>B</u>" includes all subsets for <u>A</u> (1, 2) plus all sub-sets of <u>B</u> (2, 3, 4); that is, all cases in which the condition of <u>A</u> or <u>B</u> has been met will be accepted (1, 2, 3, 4).

140. <u>Ans. (2)</u>

A subset "<u>A</u> <u>and</u> <u>B</u>" includes all cases in which <u>both</u> the conditions of subset <u>A</u> and subset <u>B</u> must be met (2 only).

141. Ans. (1)

The subset "A or C" includes all cases satisfying the conditions of subset A (1, 2) plus those satisfying the conditions of C (4, 5). However, any cases also included in B must be excluded (2, 3, or 4), for the subset we are looking for is "A or C, but not B." Therefore only subsets 1 and 5 may be accepted.

142. Ans. (4)

The subset "only" means that any other conditions being met must be excluded. Therefore, although B is composed of 2, 3, and 4, only 3 may be accepted, as 2 is also a subset of A and 4 is also a subset of C.

143. Ans. (2)

The ratio of the areas of similar triangles is equal to the square of the ratio of corresponding sides. Therefore, when $x = 2y$, the ratio of the sides is

$$\frac{2}{1} : \frac{x}{y}$$

as x is twice the value of y. The ratio of the areas is then $(2/1)^2$ or 4/1, or 4:1.

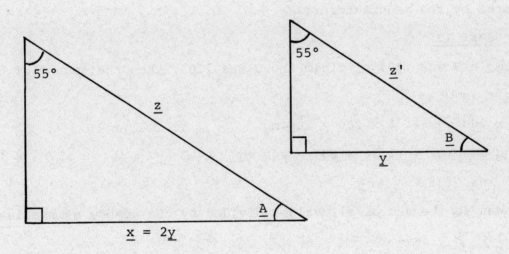

144. Ans. (4)

The sum of all angles in a triangle is 180°. If one angle is 55° and
a right angle is 90°, then angle A is 180° - 55° - 90° = 35°.

145. Ans. (4)

Since the two triangles are similar, if $\underline{x} = 3\underline{y}$, then

$z = 3z'$, or

$z' = \dfrac{z}{3} = 5/3 = 1\ 2/3$

146. Ans. (2)

The value of a bar graph is determined by drawing a line perpendicular
to the Y axis from the top of the graph. The point of interception is
the Y value of that bar.

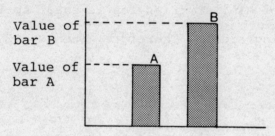

Therefore only B and C have 90% or more of the active ingredient as
declared by the manufacturer.

147. Ans. (3)

If sample B was 100% of claim and C was 120%, then the amount of drug
present is

100% x 200 mg = 1 x 200 = 200 mg

120% x 200 mg = 1.20 x 200 = 240 mg

148. Ans. (3)

The mean is the sum of all values divided by the number of samples:

$\overline{X} = \dfrac{1}{N} \Sigma \ \underline{X}$

when N is the number of samples and X is the value of each sample.
From the bar graph the following values were obtained:

1 score of 20	$20 = (1 \times 20)$	5 scores of 70	$350 = (5 \times 70)$
1 score of 30	$30 = (1 \times 30)$	4 scores of 80	$320 = (4 \times 80)$
1 score of 40	$40 = (1 \times 40)$	2 scores of 90	$180 = (2 \times 90)$
2 scores of 50	$100 = (2 \times 50)$	1 score of 100	$100 = (1 \times 100)$
3 scores of 60	$180 = (3 \times 60)$		

$\underline{N} = 20 = $ number of samples Σ of all values $= 1320$

$$\frac{1}{N} \Sigma X = \frac{1320}{20} = 66.0 = \text{mean}$$

149. Ans. (1)

The modal score is the most frequently occurring score. As five students scored 70% and no other score occurred as frequently, 70% is the modal score

150. Ans. (1)

The median is the term that is larger than or equal to half the terms, and equal to or smaller than the other half of them. In this example, there are scores for a total of 20 students. As there are an even number of terms, there exists no actual median, that is, no term larger than exactly half of the terms and smaller than the other half. But now it is possible to find two middle terms, and the median is defined as the mean of these two middle terms. In this example, if the scores are ranked in ascending order, the two middle scores are 70 and 70:

1.	20	6.	60	*11.	70	16.	80
2.	30	7.	60	12.	70	17.	80
3.	40	8.	60	13.	70	18.	90
4.	50	9.	70	14.	80	19.	90
5.	50	*10.	70	15.	80	20.	100

As rank position, 10 and 11 are in the middle; that is, 70 is larger than or equal to half of the terms, and equal to or smaller than half; and as 70 is the mean of 70 and 70, the median is 70.

151. Ans. (1)

This is a proportionality problem:

0.625 g:50::31.25 g:X

$$\frac{0.625}{50} = \frac{31.25}{X}$$

X tablets = $\frac{31.25 \text{ g} \times 50 \text{ tablets}}{0.625 \text{ g}}$

= 2500 tablets

152. Ans. (2)

Assuming that the dose should be directly related to body weight, we set up a proportionality:

$$\frac{70 \ \mu g}{150 \ \text{lb}} = \frac{x \ \mu g}{44 \ \text{lb}}$$

X μg = $\frac{70 \ \mu g \times 44 \ \text{lb}}{150 \ \text{lb}}$

X = 20.53 $\mu g \cong$ 20 μg

153. Ans. (2)

To solve for changes in y relative to x, rearrange the equation in terms of y:

$$X = \frac{1}{Y}$$

$$Y = \frac{1}{X}$$

Then substitute in the change

$$Y = \frac{1}{X(2)} = \left(\frac{1}{X}\right) \times \frac{1}{2}$$

Therefore, it can be seen that when x increases by a factor of 2, y is halved.

154. Ans. (1)

Rearrange the equation in terms of y (see above):

$$x = 2y$$

$$y = \frac{x}{2}$$

Increase x by a factor of 2:

$$Y = \frac{x \times 2}{2}$$

Y has increased by a factor of 2.

155. Ans. (4)

This is a simple fraction problem. The question is, How many times does 16 go into 24?

$$\frac{24 \text{ g}}{16} = 1.5 \text{ g} = 1500 \text{ mg}$$

156. Ans. (4)

Determine the weight that represents a 10% error. The range of acceptable weights would be all the tablet weights that are within 150 g $\pm$ the 10% error:

$$150 \text{ g} \times \frac{10\%}{100\%} = 15 \text{ g}$$

150 g - 15 g = 135 g

150 g + 15 g = 165 g

So the range is 165-135 g.

157. Ans. (1)

A percentage is the amount per hundred. A proportion should then be set up to find how much iron is in 100 mg of ferrous sulfate, knowing the ratio of 65 mg/325 mg, iron to ferrous sulfate:

$$\frac{X}{100\%} = \frac{65 \text{ mg of iron}}{325 \text{ mg of ferrous sulfate}}$$

$$\frac{65 \text{ mg}}{325 \text{ mg}} \times 100\% = 20\%$$

158. Ans. (4)

Set up a proportion with X representing the number of milligrams of compound in a liter (remember, 1 liter equals 1000 ml):

$$\frac{X \text{ mg}}{1000 \text{ ml}} = \frac{50 \text{ mg}}{\text{ml}}$$

$$X \text{ mg} = \frac{50 \text{ mg} \times 1000 \text{ ml}}{\text{ml}}$$

$$= 50,000 \text{ mg}$$

As 1000 mg are in 1 g,

$$\frac{50,000 \text{ mg}}{1000 \text{ mg}/1 \text{ g}} = 50 \text{ g}$$

159. <u>Ans. (2)</u>

If 5 ml is the smallest unit marked, then all errors are related to this unit and all readings would be rounded off to multiples of that unit; 5 ml represents the potential error. In this problem the potential error is also the percentage error of a measured volume ($\underline{X}$ ml):

$$\frac{5 \text{ ml}}{X \text{ ml}} \times 100\% = \text{percentage error}$$

$$\frac{500\%}{X\text{ml}} = 10\%$$

$$X \text{ ml} = \frac{500\%}{10\%}$$

$$\underline{X} = 50 \text{ ml}$$

160. <u>Ans. (2)</u>

The average is analogous to the mean:

$$\frac{1}{N} \sum \text{values} = \text{average}$$

$$\frac{61 + 50 + 100 + 50}{1 + 1 + 1 + 1} = 65.25 = 65$$

161. <u>Ans. (3)</u>

The equation for a straight line is $\underline{y} = \underline{mx} + \underline{b}$, where $\underline{b}$ is the $\underline{y}$ intercept and $\underline{m}$ is the slope.

Thus

$$\underline{y} = \underline{mx} + \underline{b}$$

$$\underline{y} = -0.118\underline{x} + 8.5$$

162. Ans. (1)

Rearrange the equation of the line to isolate x; then substitute the

value of the y intercept:

y $\quad = \quad -0.118x + 8.5$

y - 8.5 $\quad = \quad -0.118\underline{x}$

$\dfrac{y - 8.5}{-0.118} \quad = \quad \underline{x}$

$\dfrac{6 - 8.5}{-0.118} \quad = \quad \underline{x}$

21 $\qquad = \quad \underline{x}$

163. Ans. (3)

The value of y, when x is zero, is the y intercept (8.5). For all

other values of x, solve for y by substituting into the equation of

the line.

164. Ans. (3)

The volume of the cylinder is $\pi \underline{r}^2 \underline{h}$, where h (height) is 10 and r (radius)
is 2:

volume $= \pi \underline{r}^2 \underline{h}$

$\qquad = (3.14)(2^2)(10)$

$\qquad = 125.6 \text{ units}^3$

$\qquad = 126 \text{ units}^3$

165. Ans. (3)

The lateral surface area is the circumference of the end, $2\pi\underline{r}$, times

the height:

Lateral surface $= (2\pi r)(\underline{h})$

$\qquad = (2)(3.14)(2)(10)$

$\qquad = 125.6$

$\qquad = 126 \text{ units}^2$

166. Ans. (2)

The total area is the area of the lateral surface plus the areas of both ends:

area of circle = $\pi \underline{r}^2$

lateral surface = $2 \pi \underline{rh}$

total area = $(2)(\pi \underline{r}^2) + (2 \pi \underline{rh})$

$\qquad = 2 \pi \underline{r}(\underline{r} + \underline{h})$

$\qquad = (2)(3.14)(2)(2 + 10)$

$\qquad = 150.7$

167. Ans. (2)

The area of a trapezoid is $1/2(\underline{h})(\underline{a} + \underline{b})$:

$1/2(1)(4 + 2) = $ area

3 units^2 = area

168. Ans. (3)

The area of a parallelogram is determined by $\underline{h}$ x $\underline{b}$:

$(2)(5)$ = area

10 units^2 = area

169. Ans. (3)

To solve simultaneous equations, isolate the term in the first equation, which will be subsequently inserted into the second equation. In this case $\underline{y}$ will be expressed in terms of $\underline{x}$ and $\underline{b}$. The $\underline{a}$ term is common to both; therefore rearrange the $\underline{x}$ equation to isolate $\underline{a}$:

$\underline{x} = 3\underline{b} + \underline{a}$

$\underline{a} = \underline{x} - 3b$

Then substitute into the $\underline{y}$ equation:

$\underline{y} = 3\underline{a} + \underline{b} = 3(\underline{x} - 3\underline{b}) + \underline{b}$

$\qquad = 3\underline{x} - 9\underline{b} + \underline{b} = 3\underline{x} - 8\underline{b}$

170. Ans. (1)

The slope of a line ($\underline{m}$) is the change in $\underline{y}$ versus the change in $\underline{x}$ ($\underline{x}$ versus $\underline{y}$). Therefore the correct answer is (1), a slope of $\underline{m}$. The ordinate ($\underline{y}$ value) intercept is given by $\underline{c}$. The abscissa ($\underline{x}$ value) intercept occurs when $\underline{y}$ equals zero or $0 = \underline{M}\,\underline{X} + \underline{c}$, $X = -\underline{c/m}$.

171. Ans. (4)

When one divides ratios with the same denominator, the denominators may be factored out and only the numerators divided. It may be viewed in any of the following fashions:

$$\frac{7 \div 3}{21 \div 3} = 7/21$$

$$7:3::21:3 \Rightarrow 7/21$$

$$7/\cancel{3} \div 21/\cancel{3} = 7/21$$

172. Ans. (4)

To reduce a fraction, first determine what roots of the numerator are common in the denominator:

$$\frac{72}{2880} = \frac{72}{72 \times 40} \quad \text{or} \quad \frac{2 \times 2 \times 2 \times 3 \times 3}{2 \times 2 \times 2 \times 2 \times 2 \times 2 \times 3 \times 3 \times 5}$$

$$= \frac{1}{2 \times 2 \times 2 \times 5}$$

$$= 1/40$$

173. Ans. (1)

Set up the proportion

$$\frac{0.25 \text{ mg}}{\text{tablet}} = \frac{7.5 \text{ mg}}{X \text{ tablets}}$$

$$\underline{X} = \frac{7.5 \text{ mg} \times 1 \text{ tablet}}{0.25 \text{ mg}}$$

$$\underline{X} = 30$$

174. Ans. (3)

Convert all the fractions to decimals; then add all values:

$$3/4 = \frac{X}{1.00} \qquad\qquad 2/5 = \frac{X}{1.00}$$

$$\underline{X} = \frac{3 \times 1.00}{4} \qquad\qquad \underline{X} = \frac{2 \times 1.00}{5}$$

$$\underline{X} = 0.75 \qquad\qquad \underline{X} = 0.40$$

3/4 mg + 0.25 mg + 2/5 mg + 2.75 mg = $\underline{X}$ mg

0.75 + 0.25 + 0.40 + 2.75 = 4.15 mg

175. Ans. (1)

To add, convert all numbers to common units. In this case grams (g) is the base unit:

1000 mg = 1 g

1 kg = 1000 g

Therefore

$$\frac{0.75 \text{ mg}}{X \text{ g}} = \frac{1000 \text{ mg}}{1 \text{ g}}$$

$\underline{X}$ g = 0.00075 g

$$\frac{0.5 \text{ kg}}{X \text{ g}} = \frac{1 \text{ kg}}{1000 \text{ g}}$$

$\underline{X}$ g = 500 g

0.75 mg + 50 g + 0.5 kg - $\underline{X}$ g

0.00075 g + 50 g + 500 g = 550.00075 g

176. Ans. (2)

Express $3\frac{1}{8}$ as a fraction:

$$\frac{3 \times 8 + 1}{8} = \frac{25}{8}$$

Then convert the fraction so that it has a denominator common to those of the possible answers. Those values with a denominator of 36 may automatically be discarded, as 8 is not a factor of 36, (i.e., 36 cannot be divided by 8 to yield a whole number). Therefore only denominators of 32 need be considered:

$$\frac{25 \times 4}{8 \times 4} = \frac{100}{32}$$

177. Ans. (2)

First determine how many milligrams are being considered; then convert to grains by proportionalities:

$$\frac{10\%}{100\%} \times 360 = 36 \text{ mg}$$

$$\frac{1 \text{ g}}{60 \text{ mg}} = \frac{X \text{ g}}{36 \text{ mg}}$$

X grains   = 0.6 grain

178. Ans. (4)

Both quantities must first be converted to similar denominators; then they can be simplified and added:

$$\frac{2 \sqrt{36} \times 3\sqrt{7}}{3 \sqrt{7}} + \frac{4 \sqrt{28}}{3 \sqrt{7}} = \frac{(2 \sqrt{6 \times 6} \times 3 \sqrt{7})}{3 \sqrt{7}} + \frac{4 \sqrt{2 \times 2 \times 7}}{3 \sqrt{7}}$$

$$= \frac{(2 \times 6) \times (3 \sqrt{7}) + 4 \sqrt{2 \times 2} \times \sqrt{7}}{3 \sqrt{7}}$$

$$= \frac{36 \sqrt{7} + 8 \sqrt{7}}{3 \sqrt{7}}$$

$$= \frac{36 + 8}{3}$$

$$= 14 \frac{2}{3}$$

179. Ans. (1)

This is a simple subtraction problem. If $\underline{A}$ were equal to $\underline{X}$, then $1 + \underline{A}$ would equal $1 + \underline{X}$. The value of $\underline{A}$ does not change the mathematical principle. Therefore, when

$$\underline{A} = \underline{e}^a$$

we have

$$1 + \underline{A} = 1 + \underline{e}^a$$

180. **Ans. (3)**

Any number to the zeroth power is 1:

$$7.7 \times 10^0 = 7.7 \times 1$$
$$= 7.7$$

181. **Ans. (3)**

1,000,000 expressed in base 10 is 1×10^6. Using the law of exponents (see Answer 119), we have

$$1 \times 10^3 \times 10^3 = 1 \times 10^{3 + 3}$$
$$= 1 \times 10^6$$

182. **Ans. (4)**

Using the law of exponents (see Answer 119), we see that $\sqrt{144 \times 10^4}$ may be broken down as follows:

$$\sqrt{144 \times 10^4} = \sqrt{144} \times \sqrt{10^4}$$
$$= \sqrt{12 \times 12} \times \sqrt{10^2 \times 10^2}$$
$$= 12 \times 10^2$$
$$= 1200$$

183. **Ans. (1)**

Using proportionalities to convert the total weight after summing, we have 132 lb + 11 lb + 44 lb = 187 lb. So then

$$\frac{1 \text{ kg}}{2.2 \text{ lb}} = \frac{X \text{ kg}}{187 \text{ lb}}$$

$$\frac{1 \text{ kg} \times 187 \text{ lb}}{2.2 \text{ lb}} = X \text{ kg}$$

$$X \text{ kg} = 85 \text{ kg}$$

184. **Ans. (2)**

Simply convert to a common denominator and add (see Answer 119):

$$(3/4)^2 = \frac{3^2}{4^2} = 9/16$$

$$3^2 = 9$$

$$\sqrt{\frac{49}{256}} = \frac{\sqrt{49}}{\sqrt{256}} = \frac{\sqrt{7 \times 7}}{\sqrt{2 \times 2 \times 2 \times 2 \times 2 \times 2 \times 2 \times 2}}$$

$$= \frac{7}{\sqrt{2^8}} = \frac{7}{\sqrt{2^4}} = \frac{7}{16}$$

Therefore

$$(3/4)^2 + 3^2 + \sqrt{\frac{49}{256}} = X$$

$$9/16 + \frac{9 \times 16}{16} + \frac{7}{16} = X$$

$$\underline{X} = 160/16 = 10$$

185. Ans. (3)

The equation of a line is $\underline{y} = \underline{mx} + b$ (see Answers 126-128), where $\underline{m}$ is the slope and $\underline{b}$ is the $\underline{y}$ intercept. Therefore

$$\underline{y} = \underline{mx} + \underline{b}$$
$$\underline{y} = -2\underline{x} + \sqrt{2}$$

186. Ans. (4)

Simplify the numerator; then divide the result by the denominator:

250,000 x 0.018 = 4500.000. = 4500

4500/0.15   = 300.00.0

                = 30,000

187. Ans. (1)

If we use the law of exponents, $\underline{x}^{-3} = \frac{1}{\underline{x}^3}$. Then

$$\frac{1}{\underline{x}^3} = 1/27$$

$$\underline{x}^3 = 27$$
$$\underline{x} = \sqrt[3]{27} = \sqrt[3]{3 \times 3 \times 3}$$
$$= 3$$

188. Ans. (1)

Corresponding sides of similar triangles are related by the same ratio.

Therefore

$\dfrac{J}{K}$ = ratio of one side

$\dfrac{H}{I}$ = ratio of second side

$\dfrac{J}{K}$ = $\dfrac{H}{I}$

I = $\dfrac{HK}{J}$

189. Ans. (1)

If drug A is 20% of the compound, then drug A is 20% of 500 g:

$\dfrac{20\%}{100\%}$ x 500 = grams of drug A

$\dfrac{10,000}{100}$ = grams of drug A = 100

190. Ans. (2)

Drugs A and B represent 20 and 5%, respectively, of the compound.

Therefore 25% of 500 g is the amount of drugs A and B:

20/100 + 5/100 x 500 g = grams of drugs A and B

$\dfrac{12,500}{100}$ = grams of drugs A and B = 125 g

191. Ans. (4)

Drugs B and C represent 5 and 75%, respectively, of the compound.

Therefore 80% of 500 g is the amount of drugs B and C.

5/100 + 75/100 x 500 g = grams of drugs B and C

$\dfrac{40,000}{100}$ = grams of drugs B and C = 400

192. Ans. (1)

Drugs A, B, and C represent 20, 5, and 75% of the compound, which, when

summed, make up 100% of the compound. Therefore, 100 g of drugs A, B, and C are in 100 g of the compound

193. Ans. (2)

The ratios A:B:C are 20%:5%:75%. If 5 is the lowest common denominator, then

20/5:5/5:75/5

4:1:15

194. Ans. (4)

If this problem is approached as a proportion, then the product of the means divided by one of the extremes equals the other extreme. Initially, isolate the extreme $g_b M_b$:

$$\frac{B - p}{q} = \frac{g_b M_a}{g_b M_b}$$

$$g_b M_b = \frac{(g_a M_a)(q)}{B - P}$$

Again, treat the equation as a proportion and isolate the extreme (g_b):

$$g_b = \frac{(g_a M_a)(q)(M_b)}{B-p}$$

which upon rearrangment, yields

$$g_b = \frac{q}{B-p} M_b \frac{(g_a)}{M_a}$$

195. Ans. (4)

From the equation for a straight line (see Answers 126-128), $y = mx + b$

	y intercept (b)	slope (m)	x intercept ($y = 0$)
Equation 1	4	+3	-4/3
Equation 2	-4	+3	4/3

196. Ans. (1)

To solve simultaneous equations, express the first equation in terms of a single unknown term (I). Then substitute this value into the second equation and solve for the second unknown (II). After solving for the second unknown, substitute its value back into the first equation and solve for the remaining unknown term (III):

$30 = \underline{a} + 3\underline{b} - 70$ (I)

$\underline{a} = 30 - 3\underline{b} + 70$

$3\underline{a} + 5\underline{b} = 100$ (II)

$3(30 - 3\underline{b} + 70) + 5\underline{b} = 100$

$90 - 9\underline{b} + 210 + 5\underline{b} = 100$

$-4\underline{b} = 100 - 210 - 90$

$4\underline{b} = 200$

$\underline{b} = 50$

$30 = \underline{a} + 3\underline{b} - 70$ (III)

$30 = \underline{a} + 3(50) - 70$

$30 = \underline{a} + 150 - 70$

$a = -50$

197. Ans. (2)

The question is really asking what is the total volume used. This is the total volume of a dose times the number of doses, which is then expressed in milliliters:

$$\frac{2 \text{ tablespoonfuls}}{\text{dose}} \times \frac{2 \text{ doses}}{\text{day}} \times 10 \text{ days} = \text{total volume}$$

$$40 \text{ tablespoonfuls} \times \frac{15 \text{ ml}}{\text{tablespoonful}} = 600 \text{ ml}$$

198. Ans. (4)

This problem is solved with proportions; however, as we will be dividing the total weight into smaller units, the weight should be converted to a smaller unit to minimize the number of decimal places of which we will have to keep track:

$$0.060 \text{ g} \times \frac{1000 \text{ mg}}{1 \text{ g}} = 60 \text{ mg}$$

$$\frac{60 \text{ mg}}{125 \text{ tablets}} = \frac{X \text{ mg}}{\text{tablet}}$$

$$0.480 \text{ mg} = \frac{X \text{ mg}}{\text{tablet}}$$

$$0.480 \text{ mg} \times \frac{1000 \text{ g}}{\text{mg}} = 480 \text{ g}$$

199. Ans. (3)

This is a conversion problem, which again is easiest to solve by the use of proportions:

$$\frac{1 \text{ in.}}{2.54 \text{ cm}} = \frac{X \text{ in.}}{12.70 \text{ cm}}$$

$$\frac{12.70 \text{ cm} \times 1 \text{ in.}}{2.54 \text{ cm}} = X \text{ in.}$$

$$5 \text{ in.} = X$$

200. Ans. (1)

To divide fractions, invert one term and multiply:

$$\frac{1}{120} \div \frac{1}{150} = \frac{1}{120} \times \frac{150}{1} = \frac{150}{120}$$

Then simplify and complete the multiplication:

$$\frac{150}{120} = \frac{15}{12} = \frac{5 \times 3}{4 \times 3} = \frac{5}{4}$$

$$\frac{5}{4} \times 50 = \frac{250}{4} = 62\frac{1}{2}$$

Biology

201. Ans. (3)

The cell is the smallest unit of life that can survive independently. The gene of a cell resides in the nucleus of the cell and can be considered an organelle, or part of the cellular machinery. An organ is composed of living cells.

202. Ans. (2)

The mitochondria is the primary source of energy for the aerobic cell. The endoplasmic reticulum and Golgi apparatus use energy from the mitochondria to synthesize and store cellular products. The nucleus is primarily responsible for the storage of genetic information.

203. Ans. (2)

By using a Punnett square, we see that two Bb individuals have a 1-in-4 (25%) chance of producing an offspring with blue (bb) eyes.

	B	b
B	BB	Bb
b	Bb	bb

204. Ans. (3)

Hypertonic solutions have a greater salt, or electrolyte, concentration than do red blood cells. Therefore water leaves the red blood cells and enters the hypertonic solution, causing the red blood cells to shrink. Both isotonic and iso-osmotic solutions will have no effect on the red blood cells. A hypotonic solution will cause water to enter the red blood cells because of their higher electrolyte concentration and cause the cells to swell.

205. Ans. (4)

Copper is considered a trace element that is necessary for normal metabolism of the body. Sodium, potassium, and calcium are major elements vital to the healthy body.

206. Ans. (4)

	B	B
b	Bb	Bb
b	Bb	Bb

A cross between a homozygous brown individual (BB) and a homozygous white individual (bb) will result in all offspring being brown heterozygous (Bb), as seen in the Punnett square.

207. Ans. (2)

Vitamins A, D, E, and K are fat-soluble vitamins. All the B vitamins, as well as vitamin C, are water-soluble vitamins.

208. Ans. (1)

Under basal conditions, the liver receives 27% of the total cardiac output, whereas the brain and skeletal muscle receive about 15%. The bone is relatively nonvascularized and receives only 5% of the total blood flow.

209. Ans. (1)

Sodium is the most abundant electrolyte in extracellular fluid (~142 mEq/liter) with potassium the most abundant electrolyte (~141 mEq/liter) inside the cell (intracellular fluid). Both calcium (0-5 mEq/liter) and magnesium (3-58 mEq/liter) exist in relatively small amounts in the extracellular fluid.

210. Ans. (3)

The small intestine has the largest surface area and carries out most of the specialized transport mechanisms in the gastrointestinal tract. Very little absorption of nutrients occurs in the stomach or the large intestine, also referred to as the colon.

211. Ans. (4)

Long-chain (more than 10 carbons) fatty acids normally enter the circulatory system by way of the lymphatic system, packaged as chylomicrons. Short-chain fatty acids normally enter the circulatory system directly as free fatty acids.

212. Ans. (2)

See the explanation for Answer 209.

213. Ans. (1)

Scurvy is a disease resulting from a vitamin C deficiency. Deficiencies in thiamine, niacin, and vitamin D result in beriberi, pellagra, and rickets, respectively.

214. Ans. (3)

Squamous epithelium is normally associated with body surfaces, as a form of protection (i.e., skin). Epithelium associated with the kidney, lungs, and pancreas is more suited for secretory functions and is columnar or cuboidal in nature.

215. Ans. (2)

Chromatin is composed of chromosomes and is found primarily in the nucleus.

216. Ans. (1)

Skeletal muscle fibers contract and relax in about 0.1 sec. Cardiac muscle requires 1-5 sec,

whereas smooth muscle needs more than 3 sec to contract and relax.

217. Ans. (2)

Saturated fats have all their carbon bonds saturated with hydrogens; thus there are no double bonds. As the number of double bonds increases, the melting point of the fat decreases. Therefore saturated fats are normally solids at room temperature, whereas unsaturated fats are liquids. Complete oxidation of 1 g of fat yields about 9 calories, whereas that of 1 g of carbohydrate yields about 4 calories.

218. Ans (3)

Messenger RNA transfers genetic information from the nucleus by forming a complex with the ribosomes (composed largely of ribosomal RNA) of the endoplasmic reticulum in the cytoplasm. Transfer RNA carries amino acids to the messenger RNA-ribosome complex during protein synthesis.

219. Ans. (4)

Each mitotic division is a continuous process, with each stage merging imperceptibly into the next. For descriptive purposes, mitosis is divided into four stages: prophase, metaphase, anaphase, and telophase.

220. Ans. (2)

Since biological membranes are primarily a sandwich composed of a bimolecular layer of lipid with a layer of protein on both the inner and outer surfaces, lipid-soluble compounds diffuse through it faster than water-soluble compounds. For water-soluble compounds, the size of the molecule is the rate-limiting factor in diffusion.

221. Ans. (4)

Passive diffusion of a substance requires no energy (ATP) and will therefore not be affected by a metabolic inhibitor (cyanide). Passive diffusion also transfers uncharged (more lipid-soluble) molecules from a higher to a lower concentration gradient.

222. Ans. (1)

A large sodium (Na^+) influx into the cell results in the resting potential (-50 mV) becoming more positive and thereby initiates the action potential. Potassium is already in very high concentration ($\sim$141 mEq/liter) intracellularly and will not enter the cell.

223. Ans. (4)

A large efflux of potassium (K^+) out of the cell results in a fall in electrical potential within the cell. Potassium, in high concentration intracellularly, easily leaves the cell, whereas sodium, in high concentration extracellularly, will not diffuse out of the cell rapidly.

224. Ans. (3)

The normal resting potential of -50 mV is established by the sodium-potassium pump of the cell, resulting in a high extracellular sodium concentration ($\sim$142 mEq/liter) and a high intracellular potassium concentration ($\sim$141 mEq/liter). A negative resting potential is necessary to allow proper initiation of an action potential.

225. Ans. (2)

Insulin is a hormone that decreases blood glucose levels by increasing glucose uptake and storage by the cells. Pepsin, trypsin, and lactase are enzymes necessary for the proper digestion of nutrients.

226. Ans. (3)

The liver is the primary site of metabolism for the body and is responsible for detoxifying toxic agents in the blood. The lungs and kidneys both excrete these metabolized agents from the body. The pancreas does not directly metabolize toxic agents to any extent.

227. Ans. (3)

The kidneys remove waste products from the body.

228. Ans. (4)

All these processes are involved in the absorption of carbohydrates, amino acids, and fatty acids, as well as minerals and vitamins.

229. Ans. (1)

Bile salts are necessary for the proper digestion of fats in that they emulsify fat globules and render the end products of fat digestion soluble for more efficient absorption.

230. Ans. (3)

Glucose, fructose, and galactose are all simple sugars derived from hydrolytic cleavage of polysaccharides and double sugars. These simple sugars are then readily absorbed from the digestive tract. Glycogen is the storage form of glucose in the different cells of the body.

231. Ans. (1)

The brain does not store glucose as glycogen and must receive all its energy from glucose in the blood. Therefore a rapid decrease in blood glucose immediately deprives the brain of the energy source it requires for normal function.

232. Ans. (4)

Vitamin A, or retinol, is converted in the retina to retinal, which is a component of the light-sensitive pigment, visual purple, necessary for night vision.

233. Ans. (2)

Both active transport and facilitated diffusion require carriers that combine with the transported substance. Passive diffusion involves the transfer of a substance from a region of higher concentration to one of lower concentration without a carrier.

234. Ans. (2)

Saturation of the carrier with the transferring substance in active transport and facilitated diffusion will lead to saturation kinetics. Additionally, phagocytosis also has a maximum rate of transfer. Passive diffusion does not have any of these restrictions and normally proceeds at a rate proportional to the amount of substance present for transfer.

235. Ans. (3)

Mendel's first law, called the law of segregation, states that genes exist in individuals as pairs. The theory of recapitulation states that organisms tend to repeat, in the course of their evolutionary development, some of the corresponding stages of their evolutionary ancestors. Starling's law, also known as Starling's law of the heart, deals with regulation of the amount of blood pumped by the heart at a given time. The Watson-Crick model explains how the DNA molecule transfers information and undergoes replication.

236. Ans. (4)

About 56% of the adult human body is water (H_2O), with the rest of the body being primarily composed of organic molecules containing carbon. Therefore, of the four stated elements, calcium would be the least abundant in the human body.

237. Ans. (3)

Most species of animals and plants have chromosome numbers between 10 and 50. Humans have 46 chromosomes in each of their cells. Abnormalities in the chromosome number include Turner's syndrome (45 chromosomes) and Klinefelter's syndrome (47 chromosomes).

238. Ans. (1)

O-Negative blood, by definition, contains no A, B, or Rh agglutinogens that would cause a transfusion reaction and possibly death for a blood recipient. Therefore, O-negative blood can be given to any individuals of the four major blood types.

239. Ans. (4)

Epinephrine is one of the neurotransmitters in the brain, especially in the thalamus and hypothalamus. Both norepinephrine and acetylcholine are transmitter substances known to be secreted by the autonomic nerves innervating smooth muscle. Cholecystokinin is a hormone secreted by the intestinal mucosa that causes specific contraction of the gallbladder.

240. Ans. (4)

Neutrophils, monocytes, eosinophils, and basophils are white blood cells produced by the bone marrow along with red blood cells. Lymphocytes are white blood cells that are produced by lymphoid tissue.

241. Ans. (1)

Actively acquired immunity depends upon the production of specific proteins, antibodies, that are released into the blood and tissue fluids in response to some foreign protein (an antigen) or vaccine. On the other hand, passively acquired immunity is a result of the injection of antibodies that have been produced in another individual or species. Natural immunity protects humans from infectious diseases associated with animals, such as canine distemper. Cellular immunity deals with the recognition and destruction of foreign, genetically different cells, and may be the cause of the rejection of transplanted organs.

242. Ans. (3)

Glomerular filtration is the process by which the kidney removes most of the waste products from the blood by pure filtration through the glomerular membrane. Hydrogen ions undergo tubular secretion into the glomerular filtrate, whereas substances such as glucose, amino acids, and potassium ions are actively reabsorbed by the tubular membrane. Tubular sublimation does not apply to the kidney or any other organ.

243. Ans. (3)

Stimulation of the sympathetic nervous system increases the heart rate, sweating, and blood pressure and dilates the pupils of the eyes. Stimulation of the parasympathetic nervous system produces opposite effects, that is, decreases the heart rate, sweating and blood pressure, as well as constriction of the pupils.

244. Ans. (2)

During heavy exercise, glycogen in the muscle breaks down to lactic acid faster than lactic acid can

be oxidized; so lactic acid accumulates.

245. Ans. (3)

Meiosis occurs during the formation of eggs or sperm, where a pair of cell divisions result in gametes with only half the number of chromosomes (haploid) as the other cells of the body. When two gametes unite in fertilization, the fusion of their nuclei reconstitutes the diploid number of chromosomes.

246. Ans. (2)

The physical appearance of any individual with respect to a given inherited trait is known as his phenotype. In contrast, an individual's genetic constitution, usually expressed in symbols, is called his genotype. Both recessive and heterozygous traits are related more to genotype rather than phenotype.

247. Ans. (1)

Sickle cell anemia is a condition where homozygous recessive genes are necessary for full development of the disease. If an individual has heterozygous recessive genes for the disease, that individual only shows sickle cell trait, but not the fully developed disease. Both beriberi and pellagra are diseases associated with vitamin deficiencies. Hypertension is usually of unknown etiology.

248. Ans. (3)

Intense exercise and training of an athlete can result in a decreased respiratory rate and an increase in the size in muscle fibers. However, there will be no increase in the number of muscle fibers, since this does not change after birth.

249. Ans. (4)

Spermatogonia (diploid) grow into primary spermatocytes (diploid), and then secondary spermatocytes (diploid) after the first meiotic division. Secondary spermatocytes become spermatids (haploid) after the second meiotic division.

250. Ans. (1)

An individual with type A-negative blood can receive blood from A-negative or O-negative donors. Rh-positive blood cannot be given, since a transfusion reaction would result. B- and AB- type bloods cannot be given for the same reason.

251. Ans. (4)

The appendix, wisdom teeth, and coccygeal vertebrae (tail bone) serve no useful purpose in man; however, the pupils of the eyes are necessary for sight.

252. Ans. (3)

Graph 3 depicts a saturated reaction, as indicated by the initially straight lines for the product and substrate. The reaction proceeds to no substrate and all product, suggesting an irreversible reaction. Graph 1 shows no apparent reaction at all. Graph 2 indicates an unsaturated (curved lines) but irreversible (no substrate, all product after considerable time) reaction. Graph 4 represents an unsaturated reversible reaction, as shown by the initially curved line. This reaction also appears to be reversible, since the product and substrate appear to have reached an equilibrium. Thus not all the substrate can be converted to product without some of the product reconverting to substrate.

253. Ans. (3)

The transport of oxygen and carbon dioxide in the blood depends largely on the amount of hemoglobin present in the red blood cell. Whole blood carries approximately 20 ml of oxygen and 30-60 ml of carbon dioxide per 100 ml. Plasma water carries only about 0.2-0.3 ml. of oxygen and carbon dioxide in each 100 ml. Plasma proteins carry essentially no oxygen.

254. Ans. (1)

Only intense inbreeding is harmful in that it leads to the production of genetically inferior offspring. A limited amount of inbreeding can actually improve the genetic quality of a species.

255. Ans. (4)

This question is similar to Question 252. Graph 4 shows unsaturated reaction characteristics (initially curved lines).

256. Ans. (1)

Beneficial associations or interactions between two species of animals include commensalism, protocooperation, and mutualism. Negative interactions between two species include amensalism, parasitism, and predation.

257. Ans. (2)

Albumin ($\sim$ 5 g/100 ml of plasma) is the plasma protein most responsible for the colloid osmotic pressure. Both fibrinogen and gammaglobulin are plasma proteins that contribute to the colloid osmotic pressure, but to a considerably lesser degree. Hemoglobin is a red pigment responsible for the transport of oxygen and carbon dioxide in the blood.

258. Ans. (3)

Only red blood cells carry hemoglobin, the substance responsible
for oxygen and carbon dioxide transport.

259. Ans. (4)

Plasma cells, derived from lymphocytes, produce and secrete antibodies.
Thrombocytes, important in initiating the clotting of blood, are
formed by the fragmentation of
giant cells, megakaryocytes, in
the red bone marrow. Neutrophils
are important in taking up bacteria
and dead tissue cells by phagocytosis.

260. Ans. (1)

Cyanide is routinely employed as
an inhibitor of enzymatic reactions. Therefore treatment with
cyanide will arrest the enzymatic
reaction, and substrate will not
be changed to product (Graph 1).

261. Ans. (3)

The hemoglobin in the red blood
cell has a high capacity for bind-
ing both oxygen and carbon dioxide.
A lack of hemoglobin (anemia) results in a decreased capacity for
oxygen and carbon dioxide transport.

262. Ans. (1)

Albumin (5 g/100 ml of plasma) is
approximately 2.5 times more abundant than globulin (2 g/100 ml of
plasma). Fibrinogen and immuno-
globulins are present in small
amounts compared to albumin.

263. Ans. (4)

Whereas decreased oxygen delivery
to tissues (or a low blood oxygen
concentration) will increase the
number of red blood cells, increased carbon dioxide concentration will not. Changes in the
number of red blood cells appear
to be associated with changes in
blood oxygen tension rather than
in blood carbon dioxide tension.

264. Ans. (2)

Sweating, increased metabolism, and
vasodilation of the blood vessels
help transfer body heat to the sur-
rounding environment. Increased
muscle tone does not significantly
increase heat loss.

265. Ans. (3)

Urea and creatinine normally pass
through the kidney in the glomerular filtrate. Conversely, normally
all the glucose in the glomerular
filtrate is actively reabsorbed by
the kidney in the normal individual. Glucose can be found in the
urine when the blood glucose concentration is abnormally elevated
($>$180 mg %), as in uncontrolled di-
abetes.

266. Ans. (4)

The reticular activating system is
involved in the control of sleep,
wakefulness, attentiveness, and
behavior, but does not actively
participate in regulating the volume of body fluids. The barorecep-
tors and vasomotor center of the
brain work together to increase
the flow of blood to the glomeruli
of the kidneys, resulting in increased glomerular filtration and
formation of urine. The osmorecep-
tors control the amount of water
reabsorbed from the tubular filtrate of the kidneys by the secretion of antidiuretic hormone.

267. Ans. (3)

The axon and dendrites are compo-
nents of the neuron. The dendrites
constitute that part of the neuron
specialized for receiving excitation, whereas the axon is the part
specialized to distribute or conduct excitation away from the den-
dritic zone. Nerves are usually

composed of collections of axons.

268.   Ans. (1)

The rate of conduction increases
as the diameter of the axon increases, because there is less re-
sistance to the action potential.
Thus larger nerve fibers have a
faster rate of conduction than
smaller ones. Myelin sheaths usually increase the rate of conduction
by insulating the action potential
on the axon from the external environment, again decreasing re-
sistance.

269.   Ans. (2)

The autonomic nervous system, composed of both sympathetic and
parasympathetic nerves, is responsible for the involuntary activities
of the body. Motor impulses reach
the effector organ from the brain
or spinal cord through a series of
motor neurons comprising the corticospinal (pyramidal) and extra-
corticospinal (extrapyramidal)
tracts.

270.   Ans. (4)

Thyroxine is an iodinated deriva-
tive of the amino acid tyrosine.
Other hormones derived from amino
acids include melatonin and epinephrine. Prostaglandins are derivatives of 20-carbon unsaturated
fatty acids, whereas estradiol and
testosterone are derived from cho-
lesterol.

271.   Ans. (3)

A single muscle twitch is caused
by an initiating action potential;
however, there is a latent period
after the generation of the action
potential and initiation of the
muscle twitch. After the latent
period, the muscle contracts and
then relaxes, followed by a re-
fractory period in which the muscle will not respond to another
action potential.

272.   Ans. (4)

The nervous system provides in-
stantaneous control of a body function, whereas hormones usually
take a relatively long time (hours
or days) to regulate a body function.

273.   Ans. (1)

Progesterone is secreted by the
corpus luteum and acts with estradiol to regulate the estrous and
menstrual cycles. Vasopressin,
secreted by the hypothalamus, stim-
ulates the contraction of smooth
muscles and has an antidiuretic
action on kidney tubules. Aldo-
sterone regulates metabolism of
sodium and potassium and is secreted by the adrenal cortex.

274.   Ans. (3)

The rods of the retina are responsible for peripheral, achromatic,
and poor detail vision. Central,
color, and detail vision is a function of the cones of the retina.

275.   Ans. (1)

The rate of lymph flow is much slow-
er ($\sim$100 ml/hr) than blood flow ($\sim$5
liter/min) in man and most animal
species.

Chemistry

276. Ans. (4)

Alkanes are saturated hydrocarbons containing only carbon and hydrogen. They are usually straight-chained compounds and the carbon atom utilizes four sp^3 hybrid orbitals, forming a tetrahedral arrangement. Each bond angle is 109.5°, and the general formula is C_nH_{2n+2}; for example, when there is one C atom, then there are four H atoms, as in methane. Alkenes have the general formula C_nH_{2n}.

277. Ans. (2)

With regard to phenol, electron-releasing substituents (e.g., $--CH_3$) will decrease its acidity and lower the K_a. An electron-attracting substituent (e.g., $--NO_2$) will withdraw the ring electrons, relatively, and increase the acidity of phenol, resulting in a higher K_a. Thus a nitro substituent in the ortho position will increase the K_a, whereas a methyl substituent in the same position would lower the K_a. Furthermore, the $--OH$ substituent is strongly ortho and para directing.

278. Ans. (4)

Using the pH concept, we have $pH = -\log[H^+] = \log\left(\dfrac{1}{[H^+]}\right)$. Furthermore, $pOH = \log\left(\dfrac{1}{[OH^-]}\right)$, and $[H^+][OH^-]$ equals 10^{-14}. From these relations, $pH + pOH = 14$.

279. Ans. (1)

Hematite (Fe_2O_3) has a molecular weight of 160. The percentage of elemental iron in hematite is given as follows:

$$\frac{2Fe}{Fe_2O_3} = \frac{2(56)}{160} \times 100\%$$

$$= 70\%$$

Note that there are two atoms of iron in Fe_2O_3.

280. Ans. (2)

$$3H_2 \quad + \quad N_2 \longrightarrow 2NH_3$$
(3 liters)   (1 liter)   (2 liters)

Setting up a direct proportion, that is, $\dfrac{2 \text{ liters of } NH_3}{3 \text{ liters of } H_2} = \dfrac{20 \text{ liters of } NH_3}{X \text{ liters of } H_2}$

and solving for X will give an answer of 30 liters.

281. Ans. (2)

The volume occupied by the gram-molecular weight of a gas under standard temperature and pressure conditions (i.e., 0°C and 760 mmHg) is called the gram-molecular volume. Hence, 1 mole of any gas under these conditions will occupy a volume of 22.4 liters. Be aware that 1 mole of the same gas may occupy a different volume at some other combination of temperature and pressure.

282. Ans. (2)

The molecular weight of CO_2 is 44 g (i.e., 12 + 32). Thus the gram-molecular weight of CO_2 is 44 g, which occupies 22.4 liters at standard temperature and pressure. Therefore the weight of 1 liter of CO_2 equals

$$\frac{(44 \text{ g})}{(22.4 \text{ liters})} = 1.9 \text{ g}.$$ Since there are 2 liters of CO_2, the weight is 4 g.

283. Ans. (1)

In acetylene, carbon forms two sp hybrid orbitals and thus enables itself to bind to two hydrogen atoms in a sigma bond. The carbon-carbon triple bond, however, is made up of one sigma bond and two pi bonds.

284. Ans. (3)

The carbon in methane (CH_4) and the oxygen in water (H_2O) both form sp^3 hybrid orbitals. For carbon, the sp^3 hybridization results in four hybrid orbitals in which the axes are directed toward the corners of a tetrahedron. In the formation of water, oxygen bonds with two hydrogen atoms via its two unpaired electrons. The water molecule still has a tetrahedral shape; two corners are occupied by hydrogen atoms and the rest is occupied by the unshared pairs of electrons.

285. Ans. (2)

In chemistry, the structural formula (e.g., $C_6H_{12}O_6$) reveals the numbers and types of atoms present in a molecule. Generally, if not always, the arrangement of the different atoms can also be deduced from an examination of the structural formula. However, the structural formula of a molecule bears no relationship to the gram-molecular volume occupied by the gram-molecular weight of a gas under standard conditions.

286. <u>Ans. (2)</u>

A knowledge of the chemical and physical properties of organic and inorganic compounds is important in understanding their chemical behavior.
Organic compounds do exist as isomers and decompose upon heating at
lower temperatures. They are also soluble in other organic solvents;
that is, like dissolves like. However, organic compounds do not react
with each other faster than inorganic compounds would.

287. <u>Ans. (3)</u>

In radioactive disintegration, the emission of a beta particle does not
change the atomic weight of the nucleus emitting the beta particle.
This is due to the fact that the weight of a beta particle is extremely
small. However, the atomic number increases by 1 and is thought to be
the result of the breakdown of a neutron to a proton and an electron
(beta particle). An alpha particle is a helium nucleus, and its emission, in contrast to that of a beta particle, results in a decrease of
4 units of atomic weight and 2 units of atomic number.

288. <u>Ans. (3)</u>

The artificial conversion of one element into another (e.g., nitrogen
into oxygen) is termed transmutation. Radioactive decay can occur
spontaneously, resulting in the disintegration of the parent nucleus,
with the consequent production of one or more daughter nuclei. This
process is usually accompanied by the emanation (i.e., emission) of
gamma rays. <u>Transformation</u> is a nonspecific term for changes in physical form.

289. <u>Ans. (3)</u>

Gamma rays are high-energy x rays of very short wavelength that travel
with the speed of light. Compared to alpha and beta rays, gamma rays
are the most penetrating of the radiations emitted by radioactive compounds. Since they have no electrical charge, magnetic or electrical
fields do not affect their path.

290. <u>Ans. (4)</u>

Atomic fusion is the process of combining atoms to form elements of
higher atomic weight. Frequently tremendous energy is released during
this process. Atomic fission is the process of splitting an atomic nucleus, which also results in the release of large amounts of energy.

The process of electron capture results from the conversion of an orbital electron to a neutron, and the energy therein is negligible compared to that of atomic fusion and fission.

291. Ans. (4)

Alcohols have the general formula ROH. While methanol and ethanol are the simplest and easily recognized alcohols, glycerine is also an alcohol, even though it has three hydroxyl groups. Glycerine (or glycerol) is thus a polyalcohol and is widely used in pharmaceutical manufacturing. Sodium hydroxide (NaOH) is a base and not an alcohol. Remember that alcohols are organic compounds in which the hydroxyl group has been substituted for one or more hydrogen atoms in a hydrocarbon.

292. Ans. (1)

Hydrogen chloride gas has a pungent smell, is extremely soluble in water, and reacts with ammonia to form white fumes of ammonium chloride. It is a colorless gas, but is not lighter than air. The density of the gas is greater than 1 g/cm^3 and is about 25% heavier than air.

293. Ans. (4)

The halogen elements are fluorine, chlorine, bromine, iodine, and astatine. They comprise group VIIA of the periodic table. Note that these elements end in the suffix ine; however, this does not mean that turpentine or nicotine belong to the halogen family.

294. Ans. (1)

It can be stated that 1 Eq of any chemical is that quantity which is equivalent to 1 mole of replaceable hydrogen ions in an acid-base reaction. Thus 1 mole of HCl contains 1 mole of replaceable hydrogen, and thus HCl has 1 Eq/mole. $HC_2H_3O_2$ is the formula for acetic acid, CH_3COOH. Clearly, only one hydrogen ionizes, and therefore acetic acid has 1 Eq/mole.

295. Ans. (4)

Avogadro's Law determines the relation between the properties of gases. In essence, it states that equal volumes of different gases at the same temperature and pressure contain the same number of molecules. Hence, if one keeps the temperature and pressure constant, the volume of any gas is proportional to its mass, and therefore to the number of gas molecules. Note that Charles' law states that the volume of a gas is directly proportional to the absolute temperature, provided that pressure remains constant. Boyle's law relates the pressure and volume of a gas at constant temperature.

296. Ans. (3)

This problem requires a knowledge of the relation between the pressure, volume, and temperature of any gas. The combined gas laws simplify to

$$\frac{P_1 V_1}{T_1} = \frac{P_2 V_2}{T_2}$$

. Note that at standard conditions, temperature

is 273 K and pressure is 760 mmHg. Therefore, since P_1 = 380 mmHg, V_1 = 300 ml, and T_1 = 300 K, we have to solve for V_2:

$$V_2 = \frac{P_1 V_1 T_2}{P_2 T_1}$$

$$= \frac{380 \times 300 \times 273}{760 \times 300}$$

$$= 136 \text{ ml}$$

297. Ans. (1)

$$\begin{array}{ccc} Fe & + I_2 & = FeI_2 \\ 56 \text{ g} & 254 \text{ g} & \end{array}$$

To form FeI_2, 56 g of iron are needed to react with 254 g of elemental iodine. If there are 10 g of iron, the iron will react with $\frac{(10 \times 254)g}{56}$ = 45 g of iodine.

298. Ans. (4)

If one assumes complete ionization, 58.5 mg of sodium chloride will supply 23 mg of sodium ions. Similarly, to give 100 mg of sodium ions, it is required to supply $\frac{(100 \times 58.5)}{23}$ = 254 mg of sodium chloride crystals.

299. Ans. (4)

One mEq of sodium chloride is equal to its gram-equivalent weight divided by 1000. Hence 1 mEq of sodium chloride equals 58.5 mg of sodium chloride and 2 mEq equals 117 mg. The concentration of this solution is 117 mg/ml.

300. <u>Ans. (1)</u>

The milliequivalent is used primarily by the health profession to express the concentration of electrolytes in solution. Since Mr. Smith
weighs 60 kg, he should receive 2 x 60 mEq of sodium chloride. One
mEq of sodium chloride equals 58.5 mg of salt. Therefore Mr. Smith requires 2 x 60 x 58.5 mg of sodium chloride. The answer is 7020 mg, or
7 g.

301. <u>Ans. (1)</u>

Percent (%) means parts per hundred on a weight basis. Hence, a 0.9%
solution translates to 0.9 g of sodium chloride per 100 ml of solution.
Mr. Smith requires 7 g, which is $\frac{(7 \times 100 \text{ ml})}{0.9}$ of solution. This comes
out to 777 ml of a 0.9% solution of sodium chloride.

302. <u>Ans. (1)</u>

The pharmacist must be well versed with the different units used to express the strength or concentration of a particular drug in solution.
This problem relates to a solution of sodium chloride that is half the
strength ordered. Hence twice the volume must be supplied to give the
same amount of sodium chloride ordered, that is, 777 ml x 2 = 1.5 liters.

303. <u>Ans. (2)</u>

Osmotic pressure is directly affected by the total number of particles
in solution. If one assumes complete dissociation, 1 mole of sodium
chloride is composed of 2 mOsm of total particles (i.e., Na^+ and Cl^-).

304. <u>Ans. (4)</u>

Osmotic activity is a function of the total number of particles present
in a given solution, be they electrolytes or nonelectrolytes. Electrolytes, generally, will dissociate into their component ions, and hence
the number of particles in solution will increase.

305. <u>Ans. (3)</u>

This question illustrates the need to convert different units to arrive
at the answer. One millimole of sodium chloride is equal to 2 mOsm
of the salt. One millimole of sodium chloride is 58.5 mg. Since a
0.9% solution has 0.9 g (or 900 mg) of sodium chloride per 100 ml of
solution, 900 mg of this sodium chloride is equal to 900/58.5 or 15.4
mmole of sodium chloride. Now, since 1 mmole of sodium chloride is

equal to 2 mOsm, 15.4 mmole equals 15.4 x 2 mOsm of sodium chloride. The answer is 31 mOsm.

306. Ans. (3)

Hydrogen has an atomic number and an atomic weight of 1. Hence it has one proton and one electron, which reside in the nucleus and K shell, respectively. Hydrogen does not have a neutron. The hydrogen isotopes deuterium and tritium have one and two neutrons in the nucleus, respectively.

307. Ans. (4)

This problem relates to the concept of atomic weight and atomic number. The total number of protons equals the number of electrons in the shells. Beryllium has four electrons, and therefore four protons. The total number of protons equals the atomic number, and therefore beryllium has an atomic number of 4. The total number of protons and neutrons comprises the atomic weight of the element. Beryllium has an atomic weight of 9, since it has five neutrons and four protons.

308. Ans. (2)

Mercury forms bivalent mercuric (Hg^{2+}) and bivalent mercurous (Hg_2^{2+}) compounds, even though mercury has a valence of 2 and 1, respectively. Mercurous oxide is Hg_2O. Hg_2O, Hg_3O_2, and HgO_2 compounds are unknown.

309. Ans. (1)

HNO_2 is nitrous acid. Nitronous acid, nitrate acid, and nitrite acid do not exist.

310. Ans. (3)

The reverse of synthesis is decomposition, that is, the breakdown of a compound AB to yield an element A and an element B.

311. Ans. (3)

When a particle is oxidized, it loses electrons. Therefore oxidation is associated with electron loss. Conversely, reduction is associated with electron gain. Since oxidation and reduction processes occur simultaneously, loss and/or gain of electrons is to be expected. An oxidized particle therefore loses its (valence) electrons, which results in an increase in valence number.

312. Ans. (3)

This is an exercise in the law of conservation of matter. Examination of the equation will show that the number of molecules of the reactants must equal the number of molecules of the products, that is,

$$2ABC_3 \longrightarrow 2AB + 3C_2$$

Reactant	=	Product
2A		2A
2B		2B
6C		6C

313. Ans. (4)

The oxygen molecule is diatomic (O_2). Ozone is a triatomic molecule (O_3) of oxygen; its properties are different than those of oxygen.

314. Ans. (1)

It is common knowledge that oxygen gas is combustible; however, it cannot be overemphasized that oxygen supports combustion and does not burn by itself. Its lack of odor and color does not help in its quick identification.

315. Ans. (4)

Hydrogen peroxide is H_2O_2. The word peroxide means that it contains one more oxygen atom than would normally be expected. Water (H_2O) is the simplest molecule formed between the atoms of oxygen and hydrogen. Two molecules of hydrogen peroxide decompose via the following reaction, yielding two molecules of water and one molecule of oxygen:

$$2H_2O_2 \longrightarrow 2H_2O + O_2$$

316. Ans. (3)

This problem deals with the concept of density. Since the gram is defined as the mass of 1 cm^3 (approximately 1 ml) of water at 4°C, water has a density of 1 g/ml; 5000 ml of water weigh 5000 g.

317. Ans. (4)

The student is expected to be familiar with the different units used in expressing the quantity of a given solute in a quantity of solvent or total solution. Molarity (M) is defined as the number of moles of solute per liter of solution. In contrast, molality is the number of moles of solute in 1 kg of solvent. You should also be aware that normality

(N) is defined as the number of equivalents of solute per liter of solution.

318. Ans. (2)

The molecular weight of NaOH is 40. Hence 40 g of NaOH are equivalent to 1 mole of NaOH. Molarity is defined as the number of moles of solute per liter of solution. Therefore 1 mole of NaOH dissolved in 1 liter of solution is a 1 M solution. Dissolving 1 mole in 400 ml would give a higher molarity, that is, an increase by a factor of 2.5.

319. Ans. (3)

If you are still unclear about moles and molarity by the time you get to this question, a review is required. One mole of sodium hydroxide equals 40 g dissolved in 1 liter of solution. A 5 M (molar) solution would mean 5 x 40 g of sodium hydroxide dissolved in 1 liter of solution. Hence 125 ml of this solution would contain (125 x 5 x 40) /1000 g of sodium hydroxide. The number of moles would now be easy to calculate: Just divide (125 x 5 x 40)g /1000 by 40 g/mole. The answer is 0.625 mole.

320. Ans. (3)

Since 125 ml of a 5 M solution contains 0.625 mole of sodium hydroxide, then 0.625 mole x 40 g/mole of sodium hydroxide yields 25 g of this base.

321. Ans. (1)

A liter of pure water weighs 1 kg, if one assumes that water has a density of 1 g/ml. The molecular weight of water is 18 g/mole. One liter of pure water therefore contains $\frac{(1000\ g)}{18\ g/mole}$ or 55.5 moles; 55.5 moles of water in a solution represents a molarity of 55.5.

322. Ans. (4)

Colligative properties of solutions depend on the amount and concentration of the solute(s) in the solution. Hence boiling point, vapor pressure, and freezing point are all colligative properties. Specific gravity, which compares the weights of substances to that of water, is not a colligative property.

323. Ans. (1)

Acid and base strengths are frequently expressed by pH values. The pH value of any number is defined as the negative logarithm (base 10) of that number; that is, if $X = 10^n$, then $\log X = n$ and the pH of X is $-n$. Since $pH = -\log[H^+] = -\log[1]$, $pH = 0$. Note that a pH of 0 is not neutral. A pH of 7 represents neutrality.

324. Ans. (4)

Since $pOH + pH = 14$ and $pH = 0$, pOH equals 14. This would represent a very basic (strongly alkaline) solution.

325. Ans. (1)

As indicated before, the pH value gives some idea of the strength of an acid or base. The higher the pH value, the lower the hydrogen ion concentration. A higher pH means that the substance is less acidic and more basic.

326. Ans. (1)

Methane (CH_4) is the simplest saturated hydrocarbon of the alkane series. It is explosive when mixed with air, is the active component of natural gas, and is otherwise called marsh gas. Owing to its saturated character, methane is not important in addition reactions, but it will undergo substitution reactions.

327. Ans. (3)

Esters have the general formula RCOOR. Ethyl acetate is $C_2H_5COOCH_3$. Nitroglycerine and methyl salicylate are both esters. Sodium formate (NaCOOH) is the salt of an organic acid and is therefore not an ester.

328. Ans. (2)

Glucose is a monosaccharide. Dextran and cellulose are polysaccharides. Glyceryl stearate is a fatty acid and is widely employed in making soaps, for example, sodium stearate.

329. Ans. (1)

Rayon, nylon, and Orlon are all synthetic fibers. Nylon is a synthetic protein, Orlon is a polyester fiber, and rayon is regenerated cellulose; however, cellulose is a non-synthetic fiber.

330. Ans. (1)

Werner Heisenberg showed that when one attempts to simultaneously determine the position and momentum of an electron, an unavoidable uncertainty
in both these parameters is created that cannot be resolved. Louis de
Broglie advanced the hypothesis that electrons have wavelike characteristics, Planck is responsible for the foundations of quantum theory,
and Bohr is known for his electronic theory of the atom.

331. Ans. (1)

Four quantum numbers are necessary in order to fully characterize the
electronic wave functions; these are $\underline{n}$ (the principle quantum number),
$\underline{l}$ (the azimuthal quantum number), $\underline{m}$ (the magnetic quantum number), and
$\underline{s}$ (the spin quantum number).

332. Ans. (2)

Pauli's exclusion principle clearly demonstrates that an atom cannot exist in a state where two electrons in the same orbital have the same four
quantum numbers. This principle is important when more and more electrons are added to the orbitals of the atoms in the periodic table.

333. Ans. (2)

The student is expected to remember the atomic numbers of the first 10
elements in the periodic table. Oxygen has eight electrons and its or-
bitals are filled according to a $1\underline{s}^2 2\underline{s}^2 2\underline{p}^4$ electronic configuration.
You should remember the minimum (or maximum) number of electrons that
can occupy any orbital. These s, p, d and f orbitals can be completely
filled by 2, 6, 10 and 14 electrons, respectively.

334. Ans. (2)

Carbon has six protons and therefore six electrons; however, its atomic
weight is 12; that is, it has six protons and six neutrons. Hence carbon has six protons, six electrons, and six neutrons. Remember that the
atomic number is equal to the number of protons (or electrons) and that
the atomic weight is the number of protons and neutrons in the nucleus.

335. Ans. (2)

The $1\underline{s}^2 2\underline{s}^2 2\underline{p}^2$ electronic distribution translates to six orbital electrons. Hence this element has six electrons and therefore six protons.
Carbon has six protons and six electrons. Beryllium has four electrons,

helium has two, and oxygen has eight. The element in question is carbon.

336. Ans. (4)

Isotopes are atoms of elements having the same number of electrons, the same chemical characteristics, and the same valence. However, isotopes differ in their mass, that is, in the number of neutrons in the nucleus, for example hydrogen (no neutrons) and tritium (two neutrons).

337. Ans. (1)

Carbon-12 (ordinary carbon) has six electrons, six protons, and six neutrons. Carbon-14 is an isotope of carbon and differs only in mass (i.e., neutron number). Hence carbon-14 has two extra neutrons when compared to natural carbon. In summary, carbon-12 has six electrons, six protons, and six neutrons; carbon-14 has six electrons, six protons, and eight neutrons.

338. Ans. (2)

Gamma-ray decay is associated primarily with the emission of electro-magnetic radiation, that is, photons. The internal rearrangement of the atom is responsible for gamma-ray emission, and there are no changes in the nuclear mass (i.e., the number of protons and neutrons) of the atom. Alpha decay is associated with a decrease of 4 units of atomic weight.

339. Ans. (3)

The angstrom (A°) is 1×10^{-10} m, or 1×10^{-8} cm, the average radius of an atom.

340. Ans. (4)

The prefix pyro indicates loss of water. In this example, a molecule of water is lost from two molecules of orthophosphoric acid to form py-rophosphoric acid. The prefixes hypo and per refer, respectively, to the lowest and highest oxidation states. The prefix for the highest hydrated form is ortho.

341. Ans. (1)

Lead exists in the divalent (+2) and tetravalent (+4) oxidation states, where it is called the plumbus and plumbic ion, respectively. Copper also exists in two oxidation states, monovalent (+1) and divalent (+2).

342. Ans. (2)

The alkaline-earth metals comprise group IIA of the periodic table. Phosphorus is not one of the elements in this group. Gypsum and plaster of Paris are sulfate salts of calcium, the most abundant and useful element of group IIA. Plaster of Paris is used to make plaster and surgical casts.

343. Ans. (3)

Hydrogen sulfide gas not only smells obnoxious to the user, but it is also extremely toxic. It is a colorless gas, denser than air, and somewhat soluble in water; hence the preparation and use of this gas should be carefully monitored.

344. Ans. (4)

CH_3COOH follows the general formula RCOOH, which represents an organic acid. This particular organic acid is acetic acid, commonly called vinegar. Aqua fortis is the common name for nitric acid. Aqua regia is a mixture of nitric and hydrochloric acids, while muriatic acid is commercially produced hydrochloric acid.

345. Ans. (4)

Baking soda is sodium bicarbonate, $NaHCO_3$. Sodium carbonate (Na_2CO_3) is washing soda and is used as a water softener. $Na_2B_4O_7$ is borax, while magnesium sulfate ($MgSO_4$) is known as Epsom salts.

346. Ans. (3)

HOCl is hypochlorous acid, formed from the initial reaction of chlorine gas and water. Most bleaching agents (e.g., Clorox) acts by the release of hypochlorous acid into solution. Chloroform is an organic solvent ($CHCl_3$). Brine is the form of sodium chloride found in combination with sea water, while tincture of iodine is an alcoholic preparation containing iodine.

347. Ans. (2)

Alkenes have double bonds. This double bond is made up of one pi bond and one sigma bond. In organic chemistry there are no alpha bonds, but there are alpha-designated carbon atoms.

348. Ans. (1)

$RCONH_2$ are amides, the simplest member being formamide ($HCONH_2$). Acid anhydrides have the general formula $(RCO)_2O$, amines are generally RNH_2, while azides have the general formula $RCON_3$.

349. Ans. (3)

An enzyme usually has the suffix ase, sugar usually ends in ose, while a carboxyl group would end in ate.

350. Ans. (1)

A tertiary (3°) alcohol has all of its alcohol carbon hydrogens substituted for other organic substituents; a secondary (2°) alcohol has only one hydrogen attached to the alcohol carbon; and a primary (1°) alcohol has only two hydrogens attached to the alcohol carbon. CH_3OH is methanol, which has only hydrogen attached to the alcohol carbon.

351. Ans. (2)

Vinyl usually refers to the $CH_2=CH$ radical. Thus methyl vinyl ketone is $CH_3COCH=CH_2$. Ethyl vinyl ketone is $CH_3CH_2COCH=CH_2$. Butyric acid is $CH_3CH_2CH_2COOH$, whereas $CH_3OCH_2CH=CH_2$ is methyl allyl ether.

352. Ans. (4)

An organic acid is usually identified by the longest hydrocarbon chain, with the carboxyl carbon as carbon number 1. Changing the suffix from ane to ol would make it an alcohol and not an acid.

353. Ans. (4)

$CH_3(CH_2)_8CH_3$ has 10 carbon atoms; hence it is called decane. Nonane has nine carbon atoms, while octane has only eight. Undecane is $C_{11}H_{24}$, and there are thus 11 carbon atoms in this saturated hydrocarbon.

354. Ans. (3)

Atoms in double- or triple-bonded systems are rigid and not free to rotate around these bonds. Furthermore, ring systems have an aromatic character, and the atoms in these systems are also not free to rotate around their bonds. Only atoms connected by single bonds rotate around their sigma bonds.

355. Ans. (2)

The carbonium ions, by definition, are atoms that contain a carbon atom
with only six electrons. They are classified as primary, secondary,
and tertiary ions, as in the classification of the organic alcohols.
Since the stability of a carbonium ion is greatly increased by charge
dispersal, a tertiary carbonium ion, which has three alkyl groups, is
more stable than a secondary carbonium ion, which has two alkyl groups.
The more stable the carbonium ion, the more easily it is formed.

356. Ans. (4)

Benzene is a planar molecule; that is, all its atoms lie in the same
plane. There are pi electron clouds above and below the plane of the
ring, making it a rigid molecule with the formula C_6H_6. Each carbon
atom lies at an angle of a regular six-sided figure, or hexagon. The
bond angle is therefore 120°.

357. Ans. (3)

Aldehyde and ketones have the carbonyl (--C=0) functional group. The
carbonyl carbon is joined to three other atoms by sigma bonds; there is
also an overlap of a pi bond. The carbon hybridization orbitals are
sp^2, and the molecule is planar, with bond angles of 120°.

358. Ans. (2)

With regard to chemical reactivity and nucleophilic displacement, nucleophilic substitution occurs more readily at an acyl carbon (i.e.,
--RCO) than at a saturated carbon. Hence a compound having a carbonyl
group would be more prone to undergo nucleophilic substitution, for example, amides would be more prone than amines, acid chlorides more than
alkyl chlorides, and esters more than ethers.

359. Ans. (1)

Glycols are polyalcohols, usually containing two hydroxyl groups. These
are saturated compounds, the simplest being ethylene glycol, CH_2OHCH_2OH.
The suffix ol should remind you that we are dealing with alcohols.

360. Ans. (2)

The Grignard reagent is unique owing to its high reactivity. Its general formula is RMgX, and it is formed by reacting an alkyl halide with
metallic magnesium in ether. The carbon-magnesium bond is highly polar

but distinctly covalent (i.e., sharing of electrons); however, the magnesium-halogen bond is ionic in character.

361. Ans. (3)

Organic molecules are such that reactants must be optically active in order for the products to be optically active. The converse, that is, the relation between inactive reactants and inactive products, is also correct. However, the products of optically active reactants may not show such activity, and this is due to racemic modification of the isomers.

362. Ans. (4)

CH_4 is methane, and $--CH_3$ is the methyl radical of this alkane. CH_2 or methylene exists as a discrete molecule and is highly reactive. Methanol is formaldehyde, the former being the International Union of Pure and Applied Chemistry (IUPAC) nomenclature and the latter being the common name. Mesyl is the shortened form of the methyl sulfonyl radical and deals with sulfonic acid chemistry.

363. Ans. (4)

The Diels-Alder reaction is important because the end product of the reactants, a diene and a dienophile, is a six-membered ring. The diene usually possesses electron-releasing groups, while the dienophile (an α,β-unsaturated carbonyl compound) is associated with electron-withdrawing functional groups. Note that the Diels-Alder reaction is a reaction between a conjugated diene and an α, -unsaturated carbonyl compound.

364. Ans. (1)

Disaccharides, on hydrolysis, yield two monosaccharides. Sucrose (cane sugar) will yield glucose and fructose. Maltose (malt sugar) will yield two molecules of glucose, while lactose (milk sugar) will yield glucose and galactose. Amylose is a water-soluble fraction of starch, a polysaccharide.

365. Ans. (3)

Amino acids have the general formula $RCHNH_2COOH$. The amino acid with the simplest structure is NH_2CH_2COOH, or glycine. Tyrosine is an aromatic amino acid, whereas arginine is a basic amino acid. Methionine is an amino acid containing an atom of sulfur.

366.   Ans. (2)

Aryl halides are compounds in which the halogens are attached directly to the aromatic ring, for example, bromobenzene (C_6H_5Br). Alkyl halides are not only the saturated form of the halogen-containing compounds, for they also compose the substituted alkyl group, for example, vinyl chloride.

367.   Ans. (4)

The catalytic addition of oxygen to ethylene ($CH_2=CH_2$) results in the formation of ethylene oxide, which has the structure
$$CH_2 \overbrace{} CH_2$$
$$\diagdown \diagup$$
$$O$$

Ethylene oxide is therefore an epoxide, whereas ethylene is an alkene.

368.   Ans. (3)

Amines have the general formula RNH_2. Primary amines have the formula RNH_2, secondary amines have the formula R_2NH, and tertiary amines have the formula R_3N. RNH is an amine radical and lacks either an R group or a hydrogen atom.

369.   Ans. (3)

One hundred percent alcohol (or 200 proof alcohol) is absolute alcohol or water-free alcohol. Methanol is synonymous with wood alcohol. Absolute alcohol absorbs various amounts of water from the atmosphere and must be stored accordingly.

370.   Ans. (1)

The simplest member of the fused-ring hydrocarbon family is naphthalene, which has two benzene rings. Anthracene has three fused benzene rings, just like phenanthrene.

371.   Ans. (2)

CH_3OH is the formula for an organic alcohol commonly known as methanol. Menthone is a long-chained organic compound (i.e., a terpene) with a keto group, whereas mesitol is trimethyl phenol, an alkyl-substituted aryl alcohol. Menthol is a cyclic alcohol derived from mint oils.

372.   Ans. (3)

Tollen's reagent contains $Ag(NH_3)_2^+$, the silver ammonium ion. Oxidation of an aldehyde to an acid is accompanied by the formation of a silver mirror. The latter is the result of the reduction of the soluble silver ion to yield free silver metal.

373. Ans. (4)

Ammonia has the formula NH_3. Nitrogen uses four sp^3 orbitals in forming this molecule; they are directed toward the corners of a regular tetrahedron, with one orbital containing a pair of electrons. The other three each contain a single electron.

374. Ans. (2)

By converting an organic acid to an acid chloride, we can produce a substance from which we can form esters and amides. Acid chlorides are much more reactive than their original acid and are therefore quite useful. Because of their reactivity, thionyl chloride and the chlorides of phosphorus are commonly employed in the preparation of acid chlorides. Note that these compounds have sulfur or phosphorus as the inorganic element. Ethyl chloride is a substituted halogenated hydrocarbon and plays no role in the preparation of such acid chlorides.

375. Ans. (1)

All monosaccharides are reducing sugars, that is, they reduce Tollen's or Fehling's reagent. These monosaccharides can be aldo or keto sugars. Glucose is a monosaccharide and hence a reducing sugar. Most disaccharides are reducing sugars as well. Even though sucrose is a disaccharide, it does not, however, reduce Tollen's or Fehling's solution.

Reading Comprehension

376. Ans. (4)--The answer to this question is found in lines 4-6 of the paragraph. An intramuscular solution is given intramuscularly rather than intravenously.

377. Ans. (2)--The answer is found in lines 14 and 15 of the paragraph. There are several variables, including the answer, that affect the rate of flow of medication: gravity, temperature, and possibly the equipment itself.

378. Ans. (1)--The answer is found in lines 17-20: "When the rate of flow is critical, such as in pediatric patients or in parenteral nutrition, an infusion pump may be needed to ensure the proper flow of solution into the patient."

379. Ans. (2)--The answer is found in lines 1-4 of the paragraph: "Before the intravenous administration of a medication, it is essential to check the medication, the dose, fluid in which the drug is to be given, and time of administration against the patient's chart."

380. Ans. (2)--The answer is found in lines 1-3 of the paragraph. Bronchoconstrictors do not appear in the list of items in which adrenergic agents are commonly found.

381. Ans. (3)--The answer is found in lines 13-14 of the paragraph: "General anesthetics producing parasympathetic and sympathetic imbalance may cause pupillary block."

382. Ans. (2)--The answer is found in lines 9-12 of the paragraph: "It is important to note, however, that these agents will elevate the intraocular pressure by narrowing the anterior chamber angle when instilled into eyes of angle closure patients."

383. Ans. (3)--The answer is found in lines 7-9 of the paragraph: "Adrenergic agents such as epinephrine and phenylephrine have been used ocularly to treat open-angle glaucoma."

384. Ans. (4)--The answer is found in lines 14-16 of the paragraph. "To prevent this complication, topical pilocarpine at 1% may be instilled into the eye 1 hr prior to anesthesia."

385. Ans. (3)--The answer is found in lines 5 and 6 of the paragraph: "Ventricular tachycardia usually requires intravenous therapy."

386. Ans. (3)--The answer is found in lines 11-13 of the paragraph: "Doses of 50-100 mg of diphenylhydantoin, up to a maximum of 1.0 g, may be administered intravenously every 5 min."

387. Ans. (1)--The answer is found in lines 17 and 18 of the paragraph: "Generally, cardiovascular complications can be avoided with an infusion rate of 20-50 mg/min."

388. Ans. (4)--The answer is found in lines 14-16 of the paragraph: "Single intravenous doses of 300 mg or more produce a more marked hypotension (20-45 mmHg) and also lead to subtherapeutic diphenylhydantoin plasma levels."

389. Ans. (2)--The answer is found in lines 6-9 of the paragraph: "There appears to be no indication in this situation for intramuscular injections, because the drug is slowly and erratically absorbed from the site, besides being very painful."

390. Ans. (1)--The answer is found in lines 1 and 2 of the paragraph: "In open-angle glaucoma a physical blockage occurs within the trabecular meshwork that retards elimination

of aqueous humor."

391. Ans. (3)--The answer is found in lines 6-7 of the paragraph. The normal intraocular pressure is 10-20 mmHg.

392. Ans. (3)--The answer is found in lines 8-10 of the paragraph. Visual field effects occur eventually and only after the disease has been present for a period of time. The changes are not immediate.

393. Ans. (2)--The answer is found in lines 5 and 6 of the paragraph: "The impairment of aqueous drainage elevates the intraocular pressure (IOP) to 25-35 mmHg."

394. Ans. (2)--The answer is found in lines 3 and 4 of the paragraph: "The obstruction is presumed to be located between the trabecular sheet and the episcleral veins."

395. Ans. (4)--The answer is found in lines 1-3 of the paragraph: "Besides loss of consciousness, these syncopal attacks involve pallor, muscular twitching, and sometimes seizures."

396. Ans. (2)--The answer is found in lines 15-17 of the paragraph: "An adverse dose-related effect is hypotension, which may occur by alpha-adrenergic receptor blockade or by a direct negative inotropic effect on the heart."

397. Ans. (2)--The answer is found in lines 3-5 of the paragraph: "When an EKG is obtained during an attack, the pattern indicates ventricular tachyarrhythmia."

398. Ans. (3)--The answer is found in line 1 of the paragraph: "An unusual reaction to quinidine is syncope."

399. Ans. (3)--The answer is found in line 13 of the paragraph: graph: "Syncope may occur at low

doses (e.g., 0.8 g/day)."

400. Ans. (2)--The answer is found in lines 1-3 of the paragraph: "Many reports have indicated that the tricyclic antidepressants, especially imipramine, may be of benefit in the treatment of MBD in children."

401. Ans. (1)--The answer is found in lines 8 and 9 of the paragraph: "the maximum daily dose approved by the FDA (5 mg/kg per day)...."

402. Ans. (3)--The answer is found in lines 3-5 of the paragraph: "However, although most studies have indicated their superiority over placebos, they are still not as effective as the psychostimulants."

403. Ans. (2)--The answer is found in lines 12-14 of the paragraph: "In addition, the patient should be monitored for more severe effects on the central nervous system, for example, seizures."

404. Ans. (4)--The answer is found in lines 5-8 of the paragraph. "Further drawbacks associated with their use include the development of tolerance in some children and numerous deleterious side effects."

405. Ans. (2)--The answer is found in lines 6-8 of the paragraph: "Dextroamphetamine was initially used in 1937 and continued to be the agent of choice until the late 1960s."

406. Ans. (1)--The answer is found in lines 15-17 of the paragraph: "while proponents of dextroamphetamine indicate that, in their hands, it has comparable clinical efficacy at a lower cost."

407. Ans. (4)--The answer is found in lines 1-3 of the paragraph: "The primary agents in the treatment of MBD are the centrally acting sympathomimetics, for example,

methylphenidate, dextroamphetamine, and magnesium pemoline."

408. Ans. (3)--The answer is found in lines 8-10 of the paragraph: "Methylphenidate usage increased in association with reports of a lower incidence of side effects with the latter drug."

409. Ans. (2)--The answer is found in line 1 of the paragraph: "Procainamide may be considered as an alternative to quinidine."

410. Ans. (1)--The answer is found in lines 9-11 of the paragraph: "Giardina et al. have intravenously administered 100 mg, up to a maximum of 1 g, every 5 min to treat ventricular arrhythmia."

411. Ans. (4)--The answer is found in lines 8 and 9 of the paragraph: "Procainamide may be given intravenously at a rate of 25-50 mg/min."

412. Ans. (3)--The answer is found in line 3 of the paragraph:agraph: "Most patients absorb 75-95% of an oral dose."

413. Ans. (1)--The answer is found in lines 3 and 4 of the paragraph: "However, Koch-Weser estimated that 10% of subjects may absorb 50% or less."

414. Ans. (2)--The answer is found in lines 10-12 of the paragraph: "The increase in intraocular pressure is approximately 10 mmHg for patients with preglaucomatous anterior chambers."

415. Ans. (2)--The answer is found in lines 11-13 of the paragraph: "This ocular hypertensive effect is usually fully reversible within 1 month after discontinuation of steroid therapy."

416. Ans. (2)--The answer is found in lines 12-14 of the paragraph: "In some cases irreversible eye damage occurs if ocular tension persists for 1-2 months or longer."

417. Ans. (3)--The answer is found in lines 1-3 of the paragraph: "This form of glaucoma is usually painless and involves no ocular findings or visual field defects."

418. Ans. (2)--The answer is found in lines 17-19 of the paragraph. "Patients undergoing chronic topical steroid therapy should therefore have a tonometric examination every 2 months."